Genetic Counselling

A Psychological Approach

The role of a genetic counsellor is to mediate between the rapid advances in molecular medicine and an individual's ability to understand and manage the risks of their inheritance. Counsellors therefore, need to be fully in command of the psychological impact of their communications. Written by a psychiatrist who later became a psychotherapist, this book is essential reading for counsellors of all disciplines. It examines the psychological processes involved and uses the framework of attachment theory to explain why people approach and respond to genetic counselling differently. Effective counselling requires a knowledge of the principles from individual and family therapy. In particular an in-depth understanding of empathy enables the counsellor to help the individual contain anxiety and process grief, and so facilitate decision-making or help with the effects of having a test result. The effect of counselling on the counsellor is examined creatively in order to enrich the interview with clients and the concept of non-directiveness is discussed in the context of similar approaches in family therapy and psychoanalysis. The theme of the professional relationship and its importance is seen as the most important factor.

CHRISTINE EVANS trained as a psychiatrist and worked with disturbed adolescents before retraining as a psychotherapist. She has 10 years' experience of working with genetic counsellors. Her work includes experience as a Child and Adolescent Psychiatrist and as a Psychotherapist. Her particular interest is the integration of the psychological and physical aspects of medicine. Her present practice involves working in individual psychotherapy and teaching and running workshops on attachment theory and its use in consultations in medicine, psychiatry and psychotherapy.

Time past and time present
Are both perhaps present in time future,
And time future contained in time past.
If all time is eternally present
All time is unredeemable.

T. S. Eliot. *Burnt Norton*

**To Dan and our genetic future
Richard, Hywel and Jo;
Emily and Lowri**

Contents

Acknowledgements

This book began when Helen Hughes introduced me to the world of clinical genetics at The Institute of Medical Genetics, Cardiff. The actual production has taken a long time, crystallising the ideas and putting the work on paper. It presents my understanding of the clinical work very many people shared with me. They are too numerous to name individually, but I thank everyone who took part in the teaching and supervision sessions we organised and hope the book reflects their commitment to patient care. I have tried to protect the confidentiality of patients and our discussions by building in an element of fiction.

Some people have been particularly helpful. Peter Harper, who not only supported my work with the supervision group, but also seeded the idea of recording it and contributed by writing a foreword. Jonathon Gray and Annie Procter have provided ongoing encouragement and support at times of my failing spirit and Helen Hughes has generously given time to provide comments, phraseology and advice.

My psychological friends and colleagues have provided suggestions, support and encouragement, and tolerated my preoccupation with this project. In particular, Eddy Street, who has helped on many occasions with the macro-editing to help me find a meaningful structure to present the ideas. My thanks to my friends, Steve Bowkett, who has worked with me to improve phrase and construction and Helen Rowlands, who has the ability to detect missing links of thought. I have particularly valued the conversations with Mark Rivett, Srikant Sarangi and Jeremy Holmes. Some friends have not performed any particular role but helped sustain me.

No book is written without a considerable degree of time, hard labour and self-absorption which has taken me away from family and friends. My thanks to all but, in particular, Dan, who generously provided a safe place for me to explore my own thoughts and uncomplainingly supported me by his involvement in the many difficult tasks such as referencing accurately as well as generally keeping the show on the road.

Foreword

Conversation and communication lie at the heart of genetic counselling. How well we are able to communicate will to a large extent determine how successful we are in providing answers to the questions and problems posed by those whom we see in genetic counselling practice. We hope and believe that we are already skilful in the processes involved but, at the same time, most of us recognise that we could do much better and can think of many occasions when we have been left with a sense of inadequacy, or even failure.

This book will be of great support to all involved in genetic counselling, giving both general and specific information that relates directly to its practice. The general themes explored will be especially helpful to those many people whose training has involved little theoretical knowledge of psychology and psychotherapy. By exploring this general background, notably attachment theory, in the specific context of genetic counselling, Christine Evans introduces the reader gently to the concepts involved. As a result, one comes to understand the fuller significance of factors that most of us have already intuitively recognised, but have not been able to name or relate to general principles. As she states in her preface, 'It is a way of giving back to the world of genetics what actually belongs to it'.

At a more specific level, the many quotations from individual consultations show how often the counsellor can adapt an interview to make it more fruitful, even therapeutic, using simple ways to remove blocks or open up important paths. Encouragingly, the message is that those of us in genetic counselling are often doing this already, though unconsciously; greater awareness of these approaches will allow us to use them more systematically and more confidently.

For many years I have had the great privilege of having the author as a colleague, and of being able to learn from her directly. It gives me the greatest pleasure that by writing this book she has made her experience and wisdom available to the wider genetic counselling community. Whether as professionals or as families with genetic disorders, we shall all benefit from the insights and direct help that this valuable book contains.

Peter Harper,
University Research Professor in Human Genetics,
Institute of Medical Genetics,
Cardiff University.

This book helps the counsellor understand how the personal history and emotional dynamics of the individuals who to seek help and information have the potential to inhibit the quality of communication and emotional attunement in a counselling interaction. These delicate processes are addressed by a process of critical observation, analytical description, and psychological translation of genetic counselling. The book is a valuable resource providing a deeper understanding of what is being done well and why. It is a working manual that aids two key areas of the counselling process: namely, the counsellor's knowledge and management of self, and the development of strategies that facilitate the provision of a secure and flexible framework within which the genetic counselling process can provide for those who access it.

Annie Procter
Consultant Clinical Geneticist and Clinical Director,
Institute of Medical Genetics,
University Hospital of Wales, Cardiff.

In this remarkable work, Dr. Chris Evans, a psychoanalytic psychotherapist, family therapist, and child psychiatrist, brings together her psychological expertise with long experience of working with clients and counsellors in a genetic counselling unit. The result is a book that resonates far beyond its chosen subject. Dr. Evans shows, in her own words, how genetic counselling is more than an exchange of technical information, it is an encounter between people and about people, their pain, their fears, and their relationships. Packed with illuminating and moving clinical examples, she explores the ways in which effective counsellors create a psychological space within which listening, tracking, empathy, and metaphor can help clients make choices, come to terms with their difficult feelings, and resolve conflicts. Dr. Evans's tone throughout is wise, calm, caring, considered, and unsentimental. She has an exemplary gift for making complex psychological concepts such as defense mechanisms and attachment styles understandable and relevant to everyday clinical work. In bringing together psychology and medicine, she is pioneering the rediscovery of a lost art. This book is essential reading not just for those in the immediate field of genetic counselling, but for all practitioners who want to deepen their understanding and skills in the art of communication in medicine.

Jeremy Holmes

Consultant Psychiatrist/psychotherapist Devon NHS Partnership Trust, and
Professor of Psychological Therapies, University of Exeter, and
Psychoanalysis Unit, University College London.

Dr. Christine Evans has written a contemporary textbook that beautifully melds the fields of genetic counselling and psychotherapy. As a psychiatrist, Dr. Evans accurately conveys the subtleties and nuances of the struggles and decisions faced by genetic counselling clients. Her active participation in genetics cases and extensive review of transcripts offers cases to illustrate the stress and coping and attachment theories that she promotes as frames for understanding clients' reactions to genetic information. Genetic counselling graduate students and practicing genetics professionals alike will benefit greatly from this text that advances genetic counselling as the compassionate relationship it ought to be.

Barbara Bowles Biesecker

Director, JHU/NHGRI Genetic Counseling Graduate Program, and
Associate Investigator, Social and Behavioral Research Branch,
NIH Bethesda, Maryland.

Preface

The practice of medicine has a long tradition of making a diagnosis by building up a composite picture of the symptoms and their history, a clinical examination and specialist investigations. A diagnosis enables the course of the disease to be predicted and the appropriate treatment used. However, scientific developments in genetics, by allowing us to detect specific abnormalities in chromosomes and in individual genes, are beginning to throw light on the mechanisms involved at a biochemical and molecular level. As a result the genetic and environmental factors involved in many disorders can be separated. This has heralded the birth of the practice of clinical medical genetics, a relatively new speciality in the wide and general field of medicine. With this development not only is there is a new understanding of diseases, but also an alteration in the way medicine is practised. The availability of newly discovered genetic knowledge, to all who want it, has necessitated a shift in the dynamic between the individual patient and the professional. The days have gone when the doctor was the benevolent patriarch knowing the secrets of diseases and administering to the patient, the grateful receiver. Today, people want to take personal responsibility for their health and are encouraged to do so. There is a general interest in understanding health matters and a common desire to know about medical matters and this is validated by the individual's right of access to personal information. The individual now has choice. In particular, there is the possibility of having personal genetic knowledge of present disease, or future disease potential. In the past, most genetic tests were undertaken to determine personal risk relating to reproductive decisions. However, the identification of mutations which predispose to adult-onset disorders has increased the demand for testing and an understanding of individual risk. Medical genetics is a modern speciality in tune with today's society, upholding individual autonomy and the right to have personal information. This is balanced by an awareness that there are consequences to accessing such information, especially as it is now possible to make a genetic diagnosis presymptomatically. The speciality has taken medicine into the future and requires a revision of the definition of the patient from 'symptom bearer' to that of 'enquirer'.

Genetic counselling has emerged to respond to the individual seeking genetic information and has taken up the challenge of how the knowledge of the genetic contribution of a disease is shared with individuals and families. This automatically places genetic counselling as an educative and communicative speciality. It is practised by professionals from different disciplines: medically trained clinical geneticists and genetic counsellors who may have come from a nursing tradition or have been more specifically trained as genetic counsellors. During the process of genetic counselling all of these professionals take the role of a counsellor irrespective of their original training. This role can be likened to a translator or a bridge-builder who carries scientific information from the laboratory into the clinical arena and makes it comprehensible and personally relevant to individuals and families.

However, the information is not given as a lecture, but as part of a dialogue between the individual and the counsellor. In the dialogue there is a two-way process with the counsellor and patient mutually influencing one another. It is a human encounter and the reciprocal interactive field is an important dynamic which needs to be included in the counsellor's analysis.

The central elements of a genetic consultation include risk assessment, information-giving, decision-making and assessment of psychological coping processes. It can take many forms depending on the nature of the disorder, the characteristics of the individual or family and the orientation of the counsellor. The complexity, variety and different ways of practising are reflected in the different definitions available. Nevertheless, within the variety of practice, genetic counselling has developed a core form and structure which includes conveying degrees of information, whilst also guiding the individual through a self-reflective process. In most consultations the discussion includes the nature of the disorder, the family history and an assessment of the individual. In keeping with this, the counsellor has developed a repertoire of skills, as an educator or informer and also as a facilitator, which in combination give the genetic counsellor a specific identity.

From the examination of transcripts, where it is possible to explore what actually happens in the many different genetic consultations, a general pattern can be discerned. However, the nature of the disorder introduces a particular emphasis and this determines the particular shape and form of the consultation.

In this book a psychological framework is presented which explains and explores the experience for the individual and the family. It clarifies how the experience is influenced by the human encounter with the counsellor. The framework provides a theoretical base and a language to enrich and inform the counsellor's practice and understanding. It invites genetic counselling to use that language to sit alongside the scientific language of genetics.

The genetic counsellor does not need to be a psychotherapist, but the practice needs ideas taken from counselling and psychotherapy. To be effective a counsellor needs to develop good listening skills and an empathic understanding of the individual. The term non-directive counselling has been borrowed from Carl Roger's Person-Centred Counselling. It has been much debated (Clarke, 1991) and it is used as an ideal in genetic counselling to protect and endorse the individual's right to make an autonomous decision about personal testing.

The material presented in this book is based on the experience of working as a Psychiatrist/Psychotherapist in a Medical Genetics Department with clinical geneticists, genetic nurses and counsellors. It involved observing videos of clinical encounters, reading transcripts, personally conducting clinical interviews and providing supervision, consultation and discussion groups for the genetic counselling staff.

This book is written primarily for practitioners working in genetic counselling, regardless of their discipline and is a way of giving back to the world of genetics what actually belongs to it. However, the form is new, moulded into shape by using a psychotherapeutic understanding of communication competence and underpinned with the theoretical ideas of attachment theory. This provides a framework for thinking about behaviour, psychic pain, grief and the sense of personal narrative. To complete the picture the space between communication competence and attachment theory is filled with particular interview techniques. In so doing, clinical material and theoretical points will be plaited together to provide a balance between practice and theory.

The structure of the book can be thought of as paralleling the genetic interview, or the counsellor's professional development, in that in the early stages there are a lot of facts to be presented and understood. This can be very hard work. However, as the genetic counsellor knows, the facts are necessary to be able to progress and practise effectively.

The body of the book contains many case examples which are used to illustrate a theoretical point. To protect the confidentiality of the counselling sessions, the examples are fictitious in part, but based on actual clinical encounters.

The opening chapter provides an overview of genetic counselling, placing it in the context of developments in science, society and the individual. It explores the nature, range and components of a consultation to understand its function. This is considered to be more than an exchange of technical information as it is a reflection on an important aspect of life. The interview has evolved to help the patient address the psychological tasks required when they have genetic information. In a consultation the individual is helped to self-reflect and consider what is involved in asking a genetic question and, as a consequence, is being prepared for the effects of a risk assessment or a test result.

The thesis of this book begins to develop in Chapter 2 where genetic counselling is reframed as a psychological stress. This gives genetic counselling a theoretical basis which explains the processes involved and the difficulties individuals encounter. Stress and coping go hand in hand and both are influenced by the interaction between the individual and environmental factors. As a result, there is a range of differences in perception, approach and reaction to genetic counselling with the individual differences categorised as mature, defensive and symptomatic.

In Chapter 3 these individual differences in stress response and coping behaviour are explained by using the framework of attachment theory. This theory explains how feelings are managed differently by individuals depending on their early attachment experiences to a caregiver. In addition, the theory explains other differences and these relate to the construction of a personal narrative, the ability to self-reflect and use constructive thinking processes and includes the nature of the relationship established with the counsellor. The theories of stress, coping and attachment behaviour not only provide a framework for understanding individual behaviour, but also establish a framework which informs the counsellor's response.

Chapter 4 discusses the role of the counsellor who has the complex task of providing factual genetic information whilst also acting as a facilitator in the decision-making process. As the chapter progresses, the theme is built up of the counsellor helping the individual to prepare for decision-making by assisting in the processing of unresolved emotional issues from the past and present. This promotes a self-reflective approach to the counselling process. The principal skill of the counsellor is empathy which, by connecting the counsellor to the individual, results in the containment of anxiety such that chaotic experiences can be thought about.

Chapter 5 presents examples of how the counsellor works to help the individual contain anxiety, modify defences and attachment patterns to facilitate thinking and coping. It demonstrates the importance of resolving the psychological issues for the individual to be able to consider and absorb genetic information.

The idea of a system is introduced in Chapter 6 as the counsellor not only works with individuals, but also with a family group. The family is a social system made up of individuals of different generations, where the individuals are the inter-related parts of the system which mutually affect one another. Systemic thinking is not only confined to working with the family as the counsellor also thinks systemically in an individual consultation. The chapter links systemic thinking to the attachment theory presented in Chapter 3 and highlights that the motto of a secure family is 'collaborate to care'. The central issue for families is how they organise themselves around information about their genetic inheritance. The discussion includes looking at how information about a genetic disorder could be thought of as another element which needs to be included into the family system in the same way as a birth or death triggers an adjustment relating to the life cycle.

Chapter 7 focuses on examples of working with families and children. It alerts the counsellor to the presence of children in the consultation and how an understanding of family structure and child development can be an asset. It includes examples where there is a particular request for testing of children for adult-onset disorders.

Chapter 8 explores the influence the nature of the disorder has on the consultation by exploring four specialist areas: prenatal problems, Huntington's disorder, cancer and dysmorphology. The nature of the disorder and the implications for the individual, especially with regard to future treatment or monitoring, affect the behaviour of the counsellor in respect of the balance between the educative and psychological interventions.

In Chapter 9 the effect on the counsellor is explored and discussed under two headings: the issues which are innate in addressing genetic problems and countertransference issues. The latter refers to all the feelings evoked in a counsellor as a result of working with a particular individual. It consists of issues relating to the counsellor's personal life and those triggered by the individual. A simplified version of countertransference is presented which is based on the individual's attachment pattern and management of processing emotions, as well as undeclared aspects of the individual's thinking or feelings which are projected into the counsellor.

The final chapter (Chapter 10) returns to the idea at the beginning of the book. It takes an overview of genetic counselling, not exploring the nature or component parts but rather focusing on the attitude within the consultation. It debates the concept of non-directiveness. Historically the concept was developed to support individual autonomy in decision-making, but it has been misinterpreted and sometimes it has been turned into non-involvement and passivity or even coldness. The chapter draws on the work of a number of authors in family therapy and psychoanalysis and traces the development in their thinking of the concept of neutrality. It includes the concepts of curiosity, narrative therapy and the counsellor's position of 'not-knowing' where there is no fixed answer, but a number of different perspectives.

An overview of genetic counselling

It is tempting to begin this book about the psychological aspects of the speciality of medical genetics by focusing on the individuals and families concerned and to explore the effect or the personal meaning of having a genetic consultation. However, good medical training and, in particular, training in psychological principles begin with a wider view. It uses a wide-angled lens, rather than a more detailed focus, to explore and define genetic counselling. This means beginning by addressing how genetic counselling has developed into its present shape and looking at the context of its evolution. This sets the scene which is the context of the question of the nature of genetic counselling and how is it defined. This can be followed by looking at the range of the speciality and the motivation for seeking genetic counselling. With that back-drop, it is then possible to analyse the component parts of a typical genetic counselling encounter, discuss the function of the interview and ask why it takes its present form.

The context

Genetic counselling has evolved in the context of three different areas: advances in medical knowledge, changes in society and the basic human desire to have knowledge, to understand and to learn.

Advances in medicine and the study of diseases have progressed by refinements in clinical diagnosis and special investigations. The richness of knowledge about the factors involved in the development of diseases has necessitated divisions into specialities, which all come under the umbrella of medicine. The broadest division is into the internal or individual constitutional factors and the external or environmental factors of a particular disease. Scientific enquiry into the individual factors has resulted in identifying the gene involved in particular diseases. Integrating this knowledge into general medicine has produced the relatively new speciality of genetic counselling where the discussion is around the inheritance pattern and behaviour of the particular gene and its contribution to a particular disease.

There has been a change in society away from the idea that information should be withheld and the patient looked after. The direction has been towards the individual being autonomous and the responsibility for health matters shared between professional and individual. We have come of age. In general medicine the individual wants to be part of personal treatment plans, make a personal choice and take responsibility within the advice provided. As a consequence, the individual has become independent and free from the constraints of the old patriarchal medicine where the doctor held the expert position alone and become a partner in personal medical matters. Genetic counselling is in tune with this thinking. It exists to endorse and respond to the request for personal knowledge. Indeed, one of the central tenets of genetic counselling is respect for the autonomy of the patient. To this end the speciality has attempted to be neutral and non-directive in its stance, supporting the individual's right to take personal responsibility for decisions and actions. The challenge for genetic counselling is to balance the individual's right of access whilst also considering the effect on the individual of having personal genetic information. Genetic counselling bridges the interface between open access to genetic information and the individual. It translates and explains facts, making them relevant and comprehensible whilst at the same time making sure that the individuals concerned are emotionally prepared.

Genetic counselling is a classic example of the change in the doctor–patient relationship where the premise is that information cannot be owned by the professional, as the individual has rights of access. The question is, 'Whose information is it?' This does not mean that the counsellor abdicates all responsibility and simply hands over the information to the individual. Rather, genetic counselling carries an awareness of the duty of care towards the individual who is asking a genetic question. It has evolved to address how genetic information is given and how the individual is best prepared and supported to receive it.

Alongside the developments in medicine and society there has been a change in the individual's thinking and attitudes. We have worked to understand the basic essentials for survival and now a different exploration can begin. The innate human desire to investigate and to know more about the world in general and about ourselves in particular is advancing our knowledge base. At a personal level this desire to explore begins early in life as the child reaches out to grasp an object and struggles to move. It develops into an excitement to move beyond the family, discover the wider world and understand it. This is most likely to happen when a child feels safe and secure. It is the excitement and enquiry which has discovered the genetic underpinning of disease. Human nature is such that there is a desire to know and to understand, but it also creates a dilemma. The possibility of genetic knowledge being available to an individual triggers the question: 'Do I want to know?' When an individual has a family history of genetic disorder, there is an unsettling anxiety: 'Am I going to be affected?' One of the motives for having personal genetic information is an attempt to be in control of one's life and resolve the anxiety of uncertainty. Most people want to know what is going to happen in the future, it is a fairly common wish. In the case of personal genetic information it is possible to have an answer and this creates a further dilemma. Genetic counselling has arisen to answer the question of 'What if I do know?' Referring to the testing for Huntington's disease, Chapman (2002), like Biesecker-Bowles (1998) and Juengst (1999), is concerned that alongside the advantages of predictive testing, there is a burden put on the individual, directly and indirectly, to be tested and inform others. This introduces additional elements of altruism, duty and responsibility. Other concerns are that with younger generations being tested, people have to live with the knowledge for a long time. In addition, reproductive freedom may be hampered with parents feeling pressurised to consider and debate the quality of life and health of the future child (Ashcroft, 1999; Clarkeburn, 2000; Chapman, 2002). Wexler (1979, 1992) is concerned that people who want to know their genetic status in order to plan for their future are allowing the threat of Huntington's disease to present a block to a satisfying life.

The nature of genetic counselling

The many and varied definitions of genetic counselling reflect the fact that it is a complex and rich activity, covering numerous different types of interviews. Using its factual core, Shiloh and Saxe (1989) put forward the definition of genetic counselling as the provision of information by the counsellor and its interpretation by the patient. In contrast, highlighting its psychological core, Street and Soldan (1998) emphasise the element of helping people try to understand and cope with the effects on their lives and on the lives of their families. Fraser's (1974) definition is more comprehensive and includes not only the process of communication, but also its goals, whilst Wolff and Jung (1995) succinctly and subtly characterise the process as providing information about information. The process is more than an exercise in specialised education (Kessler, 2000), and clinical experience has validated the importance of considering the characteristics of the individual and family, the nature of the question being asked and the impact of the answer. The biological genetic point of view is not the only factor of importance to the individual as, in addition, the emotional and psychological perspective of the family is relevant.

Genetic counselling is a speciality which has grown out of the need to personalise highly scientific information from the laboratory and to translate it into a user-friendly language which can be easily digested, both intellectually and emotionally, by individuals and families. The different definitions are highlighting and directing attention to either the factual genetic information, or the psychological element and may reflect a different personal perspective or orientation of the professional. Alternatively, the different definitions may exist to reflect that the practice will vary with the nature of the disorder, the individual concerned, as well as the professional.

Sarangi (2000) describes the activity of genetic counselling as a hybrid activity between main stream medical consultations and other types of counselling or psychotherapy. It certainly takes principles from both disciplines, but it also differs from both and has established its own shape and form. It has elements of both but is actually neither.

It is a speciality which has arisen under the umbrella of general medicine, yet exploring the title genetic counselling gives some other clues about its nature. First, it is about a gene and therefore has a scientific component. Second, the use of the term counselling in the title conveys the fact that the speciality also involves a conversation, which means creating a psychological space for thinking about a dilemma. As a consequence, the speciality has three separate roots: one in scientific research, another in clinical medicine and a further one in the human sphere of communication, where a thoughtful conversation between a professional and patient takes place.

The speciality has distinguished itself from its roots to claim an independent identity and ethical framework. In distancing itself from eugenics, it has come out of the laboratory and also differentiated itself from a classic medical consultation. Whilst it may be concerned with diagnosis and treatment possibilities, its principal aim is to personalise appropriate genetic information about the risk or potential for disease. It is about knowledge and this different emphasis distinguishes it from a medical consultation such that it is debatable whether the term patient is appropriate. Indeed the term enquirer is more apt. However, in this text the term is maintained for convenience.

Exploring how genetic counselling differs both from a medical consultation and from psychotherapy helps to sharpen and define the speciality further. In a general medical consultation a symptom or sign is presented to the doctor for diagnosis and treatment; in genetic counselling (where the counsellor may be a medical geneticist, nurse counsellor or counsellor) a question is presented. What follows is not necessarily an answer, but the initiation of a discussion around personal genetic make-up and the risk of having a disorder. General medicine is about what has surfaced, therefore what **is**; genetic counselling is about what is beneath the surface and therefore, what **might be**.

Genetic counselling is similar to counselling or psychotherapy in that both involve a conversation. In psychotherapy, the process is one of a conversation around a dilemma, a conflict, psychological distress or a physical or psychological symptom. The focus is on resolution through emotional processing and cognitive reappraisal. However, in genetic counselling, there is a specific question to be addressed, which involves special information about a dilemma. It may include an emotional problem, but this is principally around the complications of having particular genetic information. Both are looking into a mirror to examine the self, but the focus is on a different aspect of the self. Both genetic counselling and psychotherapeutic counselling are about self-knowledge. The former is about the personal structural self, which may affect the psychological self, whereas the latter is about self-awareness and therefore primarily about the psychological self. Both disciplines use supportive non-directive techniques. However, genetic counselling uses a particular form of focused interviewing with specific aims; psychotherapy has a less defined aim and can be as general as the movement towards health through resolution of distress. That process may involve a complex pathway using techniques which address underlying conflicts and defences, and making conscious what has been unconscious. The latter would be inappropriate in genetic counselling.

There are times in the genetic counselling process when pure counselling is needed to help the individual resolve a conflict prior to decision-making, or emotionally process a difficult result. However, the amount and degree is questionable, and begs the question of the remit of genetic counselling. The genetic counsellor is an experienced professional in a particular form of interviewing, but the speciality has a boundary and a limit in terms of appropriate skills, remit and time. A counsellor will determine the boundary around the speciality depending on demands of the service, appropriate skills, training and personal interest. One of the aims of this book is to identify psychological techniques which are useful and appropriate to genetic counselling. These would enable the counsellor to be more confident about what is possible in a few sessions and to decide when to refer for more specialist help.

In summary, the principal difference between these disciplines is about the aim of the consultation, which in turn determines the activity of the professional. The identity of genetic counselling, and its difference from general medicine and psychotherapeutic counselling, is most clearly illustrated by an exploration of the component parts of genetic counselling when it can be seen that it is a very particular form of consultation.

The component parts of a genetic consultation

A genetic consultation covers many different aspects and involves a variable number of meetings. It will take different forms depending on the nature of the disorder. Very many conditions involve a single consultation, but others require several consultations especially where there are difficult personal issues to resolve. In predictive testing for cancer and Huntington's disease there is often a protocol of a preliminary meeting followed by a series of consultations where there are particular aspects to be discussed. The practice of a home visit is variable and is sometimes included as a preliminary introduction. It is often made by a nurse counsellor who clarifies the request, collects some of the historical information and discusses some of the necessary themes to be covered. The visit also serves the purpose of providing an assessment of the relationship patterns of the family within the home setting, as they can be distorted in the clinic setting. The preliminary meeting also eases the individual's entry into the consultation process.

Each consultation is unique, but there are some general themes which are common to all disorders and these include:

1. An exploration and clarification of the nature of the request and motivation for the consultation.
2. Mapping the path of the gene across the generations, which involves building up a family tree.
3. Eliciting an understanding of the disorder to include the family-held beliefs and personal experiences of the disorder.
4. Giving the individual or family factual information about genetic inheritance processes and an understanding of the disorder in question.
5. Discussing the management of anxiety, individual personality characteristics and coping style, including the external emotional support network. Exploring awareness of the possible consequences of having personal genetic information.

1. Exploring and clarifying the nature of the request and motivation for a consultation

In the initial meeting the thoughts and questions in a genetic counsellor's mind include, 'Who is asking what question?' 'Why now?' 'Can an answer be given?' 'How useful would an answer be?' 'To whom?' and 'What are the consequences?' In addition, the way the family disorder was first noticed, or how information about it was exchanged between family members is considered. These thoughts and questions not only focus the aim of the consultation, but also ensure that the counsellor and patient have the same agenda.

The counsellor will be exploring how and when the idea of a consultation arose, what triggered it and who wants it; but equally important, who does *not* want it. A request made by a professional may not have the support or understanding of the family or individual. These initial thoughts and questions not only clarify and focus the nature of the request, but also make clear the dynamic around the request, revealing agreement or conflict.

When an individual comes for a consultation, there may be a challenge to the family culture of silence, or it may bring different views to the surface. For example, when there is a family history of Huntington's disease there may be differing opinions between a couple, with one partner wanting information and the other not. There may be a debate within an individual, as well as between people. The individual may not be sure, vacillating between wanting to know, yet fearing it and consequently, needing help to think and explore the issues around knowledge. These different views whether in a family, or inside an individual, illustrate that having genetic knowledge is not neutral information, as its consequences are highly significant. Ambivalence around knowing is understandable, with desire and fear of knowing struggling for resolution.

The underlying motivational force behind a request for a consultation is often fear or anxiety. It may be about the individual's future health, a pregnancy, a future pregnancy, or a child. The manner in which individuals handle fear will be a major determining factor in the approach to a genetic question. Sometimes there are the obvious advantages in being tested as, for example, in order to access monitoring services for the management of cancer or polycystic kidney disease. Under those circumstances the fear of knowing can be attenuated by the benefits of early diagnosis and monitoring. However, for other disorders the advantages are very much open to a personal construction.

Evers-Kiebooms et al. (1989) explored the motivation of 'at risk' individuals and their partners in deciding for or against predictive testing for Huntingdon's disease. They found that there was a difference between the intention to take the predictive test and actually making use of it and that it was not related to socio-demographic variables of sex, age, marital status, educational level or the presence of children. However, there was an association with the age of onset of the disease in the affected parent; the younger the parent when symptoms first appeared, the stronger the intention to take the test. This may be related to the length of time the child was exposed to a symptomatic parent, or the child witnessing the progressively disabling nature of the disease at a vulnerable and impressionable age and, possibly, suffering from erratic or disturbing parental behaviour. Other studies have shown that those who accept testing for Huntington's disease, hereditary breast cancer or hereditary non-polyposis colorectal cancer (HNPCC) have higher educational levels than the general population (Lerman et al., 1996; Codori et al., 1997).

The uptake for different disorders is different, being higher where there is a possible intervention. For Huntington's disease it is 10–20% (Bloch et al., 1989; Craufurd et al., 1997), for breast cancer or HNPCC the figure is 40–60% (Lerman et al., 1996; Croyle et al., 1997) and for those at risk of familial adenomatous polyposis (FAP) the test uptake is 80% (Evans et al., 1997). Differences in gender are reported, with women more likely to accept testing for Huntington's disease than men (Bloch et al., 1989; Craufurd et al., 1989). Distress about the disease itself has been found to motivate testing for high-risk breast cancer (Lerman, 1997).

The survey of 104 subjects at risk of Huntington's disease and 58 partners by Evers-Kiebooms et al. (1989), which was supported by a similar study by Tibben et al. (1990), found that the motives of those in favour of taking the predictive test were: to be certain and to make arrangements for the future. In those still at an age to have children, the motivation was linked to making a decision about having children; for those who already had children, the need to inform them played an important part. A further motivation for a consultation can be to clarify whether any apparent signs of the disease have already appeared.

In contrast, for those not in favour of taking the test, there was a correlation with the individual being aware that there is no treatment, a bad result being considered to be too difficult to live with, or that uncertainty was preferable. The fact that the result does not predict when the disease would present created another different uncertainty. Other worries might be that a bad result would interfere with a relationship.

These different approaches to taking a predictive test highlight that there are consequences to being tested, not only in Huntington's disease, but in all testing. They are not only a reflection of the disorder, but also can be understood as being determined by individual differences in attitudes, which will be discussed in a later chapter.

2. Building up a family tree

A family tree is a map of the path of the gene across the generations and usually it is established by the counsellor in the first meeting. It provides essential information which forms the basis of the risk assessment of the disease. It also tells the story of the gene across the generations and contains details of the family relationships, attitudes, emotional climate and culture, both in its content and, in the way the story is told. The family interactional pattern is made clear and in particular, the manner in which the family communicate with one another with regard to the genetic inheritance. In addition, it is important to observe the nature of the relationship the individual establishes with the counsellor.

Drawing a family tree provides essential factual information for the counsellor and the patient. In clarifying the inheritance pattern and communication pattern for the counsellor, the patient is bringing the information more prominently into personal, conscious, awareness. There may be no new facts for the patient (they are already known), nor revelations about relationships and communication patterns, but the counsellor's questions may bring new insights or a different understanding to the facts. As a consequence a different story or understanding then evolves. In addition and most importantly, the individual may begin to think in a more reflective way.

Drawing a family tree also exposes gaps in the knowledge of family connections. It invites the individual to think about those gaps, their function, how they have arisen and whether they can or need to be filled. The gaps may exist because the family have kept the information a secret, or relationships may have broken down. Alternatively, the gap may be internal where the individual has 'forgotten' an upsetting experience, repressed it and made the distress unavailable to the conscious mind. Filling the gaps can be either a simple matter or more complex when it will involve an exploration of either the personal internal world or external world of the family. In the former, this will include resurrecting past painful memories; in the latter, it may involve the individual in contacting previously estranged members of the family. Although this task may be difficult, it holds the potential for healing feuds and resolving differences. Unfortunately, that is not always possible as the exploration involves opening up of old wounds and these may carry too much hurt to be repaired.

A family tree is a review of the whole family: it brings the whole family into the room. Even in an individual consultation the family is always in the room, carried by the individual, contained in the body and mind, and expressed in behaviour and emotional expression. The family and the individual are both contained in every consultation. The family history contains facts and experiences, covering genetic aspects and psychological experiences and these are expressed, or contained, in the individual's words and physical and psychological make-up. The consultation involves revisiting and exploring the past, looking at the present and projecting into the future. The past, present and future are present in the individual at the same time and this is the focus of the discussion. So, for the individual, it is, 'This is how things have been in my family', 'What does that give me?' and 'How will I be in the future?'

3. Eliciting the individual's understanding of the disorder

Before giving any information the genetic counsellor explores what is already understood about the disorder in question. This question uncovers the accuracy of the individual's knowledge of the disorder and also the level of understanding about genetic inheritance patterns across the generations. This factual knowledge will carry the personal experience gleaned from living with an affected parent, or knowing of an affected relative. It will uncover not only painful personal experiences, but also the communication patterns of how the information was shared, the family coping pattern and the family mythology of what sense they have made of their genetic inheritance. The family mythology is the story the family have constructed to understand and give meaning to their lives (Byng-Hall, 1995a). In genetic counselling it is not surprising to find that the family mythology is often different from the objective genetic reality of the counsellor.

4. Giving factual information

A central element in a genetic consultation is the exchange of technical information. In the early stages of the consultation the information is educational. It includes the general principles of genetic inheritance patterns and mechanisms, as well as the information which is specific to the condition in question. Sometimes, it is difficult to take in new information under stressful conditions. Research with patients being tested for cervical cancer has indicated that when the information was consistent with coping style, the stress levels were lower. 'Information seekers' were less aroused with more preparatory information and 'information avoiders' were less aroused with less preparatory information (Miller and Morgan, 1983).

Later in the counselling process, the information given to the patient is the genetic information of the personal risk assessment, or a test result. The counsellor knows that it cannot be given in any standardised manner, but has to be personally tailored to meet the particular request and also take into account the individual's psychological profile and coping style. All the facts gathered through the consultation will be furnishing the counsellor with an assessment of the individual which will be giving the counsellor clues about how to give the technical information. When the counsellor has to tell the patient that they do indeed carry the problem gene, it is often referred to as 'giving bad news'. The whole consultation builds up to that point but giving good or bad news is in the context of a detailed consultation and assessment, and contained within an established professional relationship.

5. Discussing psychological profile

A psychological profile is built up which furnishes the counsellor with important information about how the individual is likely to cope under the stress of genetic knowledge. It addresses resilience, coping style and whether these will successfully sustain and provide the support needed. The discussion will possibly include previous experience of stressful events and their management by the individual. In addition, it is useful to know the family's reaction to its genetic potential or history, and whether the individual has found that helpful or not. In the Huntington's disease protocol, the counsellor may suggest to the individual that they imagine taking different decisions or having different test results. This exercise helps the individual mentally rehearse the different scenarios and explore and consider their possible future reactions. In this way the counsellor is helping the individual prepare to confront any future anxiety or grief. Soldan et al. (2000) refer to this technique as 'stress inoculation'. Personal resources are important and sometimes the external support of family or friends is invaluable at times of stress. This idea is used in Huntington's disease where it is suggested that the individual is accompanied for the test result and brings a family member or a friend as a support.

The range of genetic counselling

The range of discussions in genetic counselling is vast and is a product of the number of genetically determined conditions, the nature of the request, the individual or family, the counsellor and the stage of the counselling process. Some requests are outside the diagnosis or explanation of genetic disorders.

The request may involve making a clinical diagnosis of a disorder which is already presenting and, in that sense, is no different from a general medical consultation. Alternatively, the request may be to confirm that a diagnosis, which has already been established, is genetically determined and to give further information about its meaning and consequences. The problem may have arisen in the context of a family history or de novo, but both will need to be explained.

A large percentage of consultations are about risk assessment. Sarangi et al. (2003) have identified two risks: the one of *knowing* and the other of *having*, and both these are considered in a consultation. The speciality of medical genetics is developing quickly and the number of diseases which are linked to a gene is increasing. This means that there will be an increasing number of diseases where it will be possible to test healthy individuals predictively. This presents individuals with a dilemma of either knowing their future potential in terms of disease, or, remaining uncertain. In some disorders, such as polycystic kidney disease or the familial cancers, there are advantages in genetic detection in the pre-illness phase of diseases. It enables monitoring programmes to be implemented which can identify early signs of the disease to be accessed and, consequently, instigate potentially life-saving early treatment.

Other requests to a medical genetic department include a number of issues around the prenatal period. A couple, where there is a known history of a genetic disorder in one of them, may want to discuss their future fertility possibilities. There may have been a problem in a previous pregnancy with a need to clarify the risk for any future pregnancies. Carrier testing to identify unaffected individuals is possible and this clarifies how being a carrier could affect a future pregnancy. The request may involve explanation of the meaning of a foetal abnormality picked up in antenatal screening and whether testing of the foetus is appropriate. These consultations are difficult as they sometimes challenge a couple to consider the future of the pregnancy.

Other consultations in a genetic clinic involve making a diagnosis in dysmorphology to explain facial difference and establishing whether there are developmental problems or abnormalities in other organs, when further action will be necessary.

The function of the consultation

A genetic consultation is therefore more than an exchange of technical information. It is also a human encounter, between people and about people, their pain, their fears and their relationships. At first sight the questions appear to be designed to give the counsellor information, but they are mainly designed to prepare the individual. This is done by reviewing the individual's personal and family history, considering personal motivation and awareness of the consequences of knowledge and ways of coping. The questions are designed to facilitate decision-making. In addition, a considerable degree of emotional processing takes place in a consultation as a result of resurrecting the past, or dealing with a present difficulty, or further, as a consequence of having a test result. The interview can be seen as having evolved to help the patient address the psychological tasks of having genetic information. Soldon et al. (2000), in discussing pre-test interviewing for Huntington's disease, consider the process of genetic counselling to include: clarification of what the individual already knows, consideration of awareness of the impact of the result, education to correct and extend understanding, and reflection concerning the outcome of the education.

The received wisdom in genetic counselling is that this detailed consultation facilitates decision-making and is also a very important preparation for receiving a test result. Occasionally, the counselling process is challenged by an individual who wants testing without going through the process, seeing the consultation as an obstacle which is interfering with their right to information. The counsellor usually succeeds in reassuring and explaining that the counsellor is not a guardian of the individual's right to personal genetic knowledge, nor is the consultation a series of hoops the individual has to jump through. In genetic counselling the individual's autonomy and personal agency is considered to be paramount. Clinical experience has confirmed that going through the consultation with a counsellor allows confusion to be addressed and gives time to reflect on the decision.

The consultation is designed to give information not only about genetic processes and the disorder in question, but also to bring self-knowledge to the forefront of the individual's mind. Where as it might initially appear that it is the counsellor who is asking – 'Does this person want this information?' and 'Is this person prepared?' and further, 'Can this person cope?' – in reality the function of the consultation is for the individual who is asking, 'Do I want this information?', 'Am I prepared?' and 'Can I cope?'

The consultation offers an opportunity to think about the possibility of having information with the option of deciding either way and in a sense the counsellor is protecting the individual from making a precipitous decision which might be regretted.

The counsellor's task is to cover all the various elements in one or more consultations, not necessarily in a particular order, as the emphasis will be determined by the disorder and the individual. Nevertheless, there is a pattern in the course of the consultation with the overall thrust being for the individual to explore wanting to move from a state of innocence, not knowing, to a state of awareness of personal genetic make-up. It is as if the counsellor acts as a guide helping the patient move along a pathway from one step to another.

The title genetic counselling conveys a considerable amount. Certainly at times the counsellor uses skills taken from the psychotherapeutic type of counselling. Considering the words 'counselling' in a more literal sense, the meaning is to offer someone counsel. That has the connotation of advising, where different opinions can be considered when a difficult problem has to be considered, or an important decision made. Genetic counselling can take many forms, but an underlying common denominator is the non-directive attitude of the counsellor who holds firmly to the belief in the autonomy of the individual, respecting whatever decision the individual arrives at. At one level genetic counselling is far removed from advising, yet inherent in the genetic counselling process, there is advice, sometimes undeclared, but at other times overt. The message is to think very carefully before embarking on a testing programme. In this instance, the word 'to think' means to consider, to contemplate and to self-reflect, indicating that genetic counselling involves an in-depth processing which covers all aspects of the problem.

This chapter has presented an overview of genetic counselling, exploring its roots, identity and structure or form. As with any consultation, in any speciality, the structure provides the background framework and within that the clinician can take the freedom to emphasise, refocus or deflect. This freedom comes from the recognition that a request for a consultation may appear to be a particular question, but the experienced genetic counsellor regards the question as an entry point to a discussion. It can be useful to consider a patient's question as a parcel which needs to be unwrapped, the contents of which need careful exploration.

Summary points

Genetic counselling has arisen in the context of advances in medical knowledge, changes in society and the basic human desire to have knowledge to understand and learn.

Genetic counselling has roots in science, general medicine and communication, but it is neither of these, nor is it a summation of these disciplines. It is unique in that it is about knowledge and involves a particular form of interviewing.

A typical interview has a number of component parts which are designed to fulfil the function of facilitating decision-making and preparing the individual for information of risk assessment or a test result.

2

The psychological processes underlying genetic counselling

The previous chapter clarified that although every genetic counselling consultation is unique, there is, nevertheless, a definite and general form to a consultation. This has evolved from clinical experience and is designed to help the individual address the issues involved. This thoughtful and measured approach applies to a single consultation, as much as it does to a series in predictive testing. The pace of genetic counselling protects the individual from rushing into testing recognising that there are implications to having personal genetic knowledge. This chapter explains how genetic counselling is a psychological challenge, which emanates from the interaction between the nature of genetics and the individual. There is a challenge which is innate in addressing genetic issues, but the individual perception is a key factor in determining whether the challenge is experienced as a stress. This in turn governs how the individual approaches and responds to genetic counselling.

Uncertainty and the effects of knowledge

Uncertainty is part of every day life experience, a normal anxiety about what might happen in the future. This is always the unknown territory of the imagination onto which the individual projects long-standing personal ideas and attitudes. When there is a genetically determined illness in a family, this existential anxiety may become exacerbated and the fear then becomes focused on the unpredictable genetic element of the illness. Some people will project their good luck and certainty that they are free from the genetic change, or that they will not be affected by illness. In contrast, others will project their fearful fantasies and dread of illness. Having a genetic history changes the existential worry of the future unknown into an uncertainty about the family experience of illness. This is the focus of the consultation – an assessment of the individual risk of what is certain and what remains uncertain.

Living with uncertainty of personal genetic inheritance is an enormous challenge to the individual and can lead to the experience of stress (Lerman et al., 1995) and individuals deal with this in different ways. Women at risk of breast cancer from their family histories have high levels of distress (Kash et al., 1992) and some have an exaggerated perception of their risk (Lerman et al., 1994).

The speciality of medical genetics exists because one of the ways of dealing with uncertainty is to search for more information. It can help the individual to clarify, explain and to know. It fulfils a human need to try and understand, or in every day language 'to get one's mind round it'. Learning that one will develop a life threatening disorder may out weigh the benefits of uncertainty reduction. The extent to which the reduction in uncertainty outweighs the threat of the disease depends on the interaction between the individual and the nature of the disease (Baum et al., 1997). In a study by Codori and Brandt (1994) of Huntington's disease, knowing one's risk was thought to be helpful regardless of the result, but research has shown that reactions to testing are complex and whilst positive results are stressful, negative results are not always associated with stress reduction (Lerman et al., 1991).

Researchers have explored the effects of genetic counselling and the large number of studies published is an indicator of the professional concern and expectation of difficulties and an acknowledgement that genetic counselling is of considerable significance to the individual. Most of the research has been into the results of testing for Huntington's disease. There are conflicting thoughts and answers which may be explained by the composition of the group, the addition of counselling and the method of examination, with different results emerging from the use of questionnaires and direct interviewing. Kessler (1987) has expressed concern about the possibility of serious psychological reactions. In contrast, in a large study, Wiggins et al. (1992) suggested that predictive testing may maintain or improve the psychological well being of many people, but that the overall response did not take into account individual responses. Most of the evidence is that carriers and non-carriers differ significantly in their psychological adjustments in the short term, but not in the long term (Meiser and Dunn, 2000). In other studies for carriers, psychological adjustment remains the same (Codori et al., 1997; Tibben et al., 1997) but one study found an increase in hopelessness (Tibben et al., 1992) which is of concern because of its relationship to suicide (Farrer, 1986). Further, Meissen et al. (1988) found that moderate to severe depression was linked to disease threat. For non-carriers, psychological adjustment either tends to be the same or improves after a result (Codori and Brandt, 1994; Tibben et al., 1997). In another study Tibben et al. (1990) reported on a 1-year follow-up of 18 people after presymptomatic testing. In 8 of the non-carriers the expected relief was replaced by persistent guilt and depression; 6 avoided contact with siblings; 2 of them did not tell their siblings of their result and 5 of the 8 remained preoccupied with the threat of the disease.

In a review of adult-onset disorders, Meiser et al. (2000) commented that there is limited data on the impact of testing for the hereditary cancers. One study of hereditary breast-ovarian cancer showed a reduction in depressive symptoms in non-carriers compared to carriers and those who declined testing, but carriers showed no increase in depressive symptoms (Lerman et al., 1996). Croyle et al. (1997) found that women experience significantly different levels of psychological distress following BRCA1 mutation testing as a function of their test results. Those who had never experienced cancer or surgery, and were found to carry the mutation, showed the highest distress following testing. In a study of 200 patients undergoing testing for hereditary non-polyposis colon cancer, 24% were found to have symptoms of depression. The finding was linked to being female, having less formal education and fewer social contacts. High anxiety was linked to a younger age, less formal education, local-regional stage of disease and fewer social contacts (Vernon et al., 1997).

Predictors for adverse psychological responses in Huntington's disease are high levels of psychological distress prior to the test, being married, childless or being close to the estimated age of disease onset (Codori et al., 1997; Lerman et al., 1998).

Uncertainty can never be eliminated and genetic counselling does not necessarily have all the answers; it has an answer to a particular question of risk. Even if the individual is given an answer which confirms the presence of the gene, then the uncertainty shifts from an anxiety about the possibility of having the illness, to the uncertainty of when and sometimes, how the illness might present.

In the following extract of a consultation the counsellor and patient are discussing what is certain. It reveals that the two have a different understanding of uncertainty.

Extract

A young woman attended the genetic clinic for the result of her testing, restating, 'I'd like to know'. The counsellor explained that her disorder was a result of change in the cytoplasmic mitochondria and that the change was not universal through the body, but unevenly and unpredictably distributed. The counsellor explained, by taking a blood sample all you can really say is, 'yes it's there', or 'no, it's not' but it doesn't tell you whether it's just a trace of it or a lot ... or to what extent it will cause problems .... But it's the only sort of information we can give you, we can't tell you what sort of dose you will have around different parts of the body.

The woman responded, 'Right, I know now. I'm quite happy', 'It's just not knowing it is .... It's just not knowing'.

The counsellor attempted to make sure the patient had understood the incompleteness of the information and the uncertainty which still lay ahead by answering, 'But you say "not knowing" but I suppose what I have been trying to say is, we still don't know'.

She responded 'But you know there's some' and the counsellor replied, 'So we have answered the only question we can answer'.

The patient concluded, 'But I know it's there' which the counsellor confirmed, 'Right' and the patient left saying, 'I'm happy now'.

This extract reveals a difference in the understanding of uncertainty between the counsellor and patient and as a result the two had different aims. The patient had a personal experience of anxiety, had one question and wanted that settled. Her main anxiety and her only question had been about her having any form of the disorder; 'having or not having' in black or white with no room for any grey areas. Once she had that answer, she experienced some kind of relief and could not think about another uncertainty, that of 'how much' she might be affected. In her framework she had settled the uncertainty and did not appear to be disturbed by the result, or the future uncertainty. The counsellor, however, had another agenda – that of making sure she had a full understanding of the meaning of her result. The educative endeavour was to make sure the patient had understood what had been clarified, and, what remained uncertain. At that point in time, the patient was not able to be open to any further discussion. The patient was intent on settling her anxiety which, for the moment, was focused on having or not having.

Unlike a definitive diagnosis, genetic information is probabilistic and uncertain (Lerman, 1997), and predates the appearance of the illness creating a pre-illness phase to the natural history, which is about knowledge and the management of uncertainty. This makes the speciality a distinct entity. The difference can be seen by examining Rolland's (1984) typology which addresses how the psychological and psychosocial demands of any illness are interwoven into the stage of the family life cycle. This results in acute, chronic and terminal stages of an illness becoming more or less challenging, depending on the age of the individual. Genetic counselling is outside this schema.

Historically, genetic counselling has moved from eugenics towards a psychological paradigm (Kessler, 1980) with the decision-making process and endorsement of personal autonomy being the trademark of the modern form of the speciality. However, the price of freedom of personal autonomy is the burden of responsibility for one's actions.

Genetic counselling involves a number of issues and Horowitz et al. (2001) consider the two psychological tasks to be decision-making and coping with the consequences and that these are different themes.

The thoughts inside the individual are:

'My family has this disorder.'

'I am worried I might have it.'

'Do I want to know whether I have it?'

'Shall I ask for information?'

'What will knowing be like?'

'Shall I be tested?'

'What will that mean?'

'Can I cope?'

There is an internal debate, with varying degrees of conflict which depends on the individual perception of the dilemma and whether knowing will be considered an advantage or disadvantage. Individuals confronted by the same dilemma will view the situation through the lens of their personal experience and belief systems about the world. In principle, decisions are easy to make if there are positive and negative options; choosing the positive is easy, and there is no disappointment at the loss of the negative option. It becomes less easy if there are two positive options where there will be certain disappointment at the loss of one good option, and extremely difficult when neither option is pleasant. The decisions in genetics are complicated as there are advantages and disadvantages in having personal genetic information. Sometimes there are obvious advantages in that knowing can allow the individual to plan for the future, initiate monitoring of health, or inform the next generation in order to prepare them. However, the knowledge can also be a disadvantage as it brings the fearsome reality of having the genetic potential for a disease into sharp focus, and that may bring varying degrees of fear, loss and conflict. These emotions can complicate the decision-making process (Janis and Mann, 1977). However, anxiety is not totally unhelpful, but it needs to be at an optimum level to solve a problem. There needs to be enough anxiety to be concerned and to trigger the desire to resolve the dilemma. Shiloh (1996) uses conflict theory to explain that too little, or too much anxiety, will interfere with the individual's ability to make a decision. For example, in a study of the behaviour of women at increased risk of breast cancer, Lerman et al. (1991) found that many women did not adhere to screening guide lines and considered that the behaviour was related to the anxiety provoking nature of screening.

However, anxiety is not the only emotion raised in decision-making. Resolving conflict by making a decision is choosing and that results in an inevitable loss of the option not taken. As explained earlier, the degree of resultant loss or disappointment will depend on the issue involved, the individual perception of it being positive or negative and the nature of the unselected alternative.

Understanding the potential for anxiety and loss in a genetic process is particularly important and part of the counsellor's role may involve helping individuals with these emotions, which would otherwise interrupt the decision-making process.

An explanation of the concept of psychological stress will provide a theoretical framework for understanding how these emotions arise from the challenge in genetic counselling and further it will inform and support the counsellor's response and clinical management.

The concept of psychological stress in genetic counselling

The potential for psychological stress to be experienced exists when an individual is challenged or is under a demand to change or adjust. The demand may originate in the external environment or within the individual and the change may good or bad. The adjustment process requires the individual to resolve the issue by acknowledging, processing, accepting and adapting to the changes. Stress is not simply in the environment as it is not the event, nor is it inside the individual. It occurs as a result of an interaction between the individual and the environment (Folkman, 1984) and is therefore contextual (Street, 1994). The individual appraisal determines whether the situation is stressful and the determining factor is whether the individual considers that the situation is beyond personal resources and a danger to personal well-being.

Although stress is interactional, in general, there are classic situations which have the potential to be stressful and Engel (1962) has described three main categories of stress:

1. Injury or threat of injury involving notions of pain and mutilation, whether actual or threatened.
2. Loss, or threat of loss, of 'psychic objects' such as personal relationships, prestige, body functions or image, social roles, job, valued possessions or indeed anything or person which is experienced as 'part of themselves'.
3. Frustration.

Using this framework and applying it to the process of genetic counselling, it is clear all three categories of stress – threat, loss and frustration – could be involved, but it is dependent on the individual's perception. When the appraisal is that the situation is not stressful, it will be relatively easy to proceed with genetic counselling. In contrast, when it is considered to be stressful, a secondary appraisal of coping is needed.

The following explores how genetic counselling has the potential for being experienced as stressful.

The threat

The main emotion experienced under threat is fear or anxiety. The possibility of illness in the future is a frightening prospect and, depending on the nature of the illness, there can be an expectation of pain, a changed body, or disfigurement, or even death. Addressing the personal inheritance of these frightening prospects is a challenge to the strength or weakness of the personal sense of self. There may be no physical injury, but there is the threat of being different which may injure the sense of self-integrity and requires the individual to review beliefs about the present, as well as the future self. There is the potential for destabilising the previously held self-image, no matter what the result. In addition there is the possibility that the individual's sense of personal security may be compromised. In his thesis on Huntington's disease, Tibben (1993) views the process of genetic counselling as a threat and considers that having genetic knowledge is a potentially distressing event, outside the usual human experience. He considers the knowledge to be perceived as a threat to one's life, one's physical integrity, or to one's children and may also involve social stigmatisation. Wexler (1979) considers that lack of control and fear of being overwhelmed are the two stressors of Huntington's disease. The opinion of Horowitz et al. (2001) is that the emotional distress may be worthwhile, but it may be intense or prolonged and so cause other problems.

When the threat involves a longed-for child and the genetic investigation is about fertility or the possibility of a child being born with abnormalities, considerable anxiety is raised as the threat is of a particular nature. Children are the future, an expression of the adult's immortal self and usually create a good sense of ongoing life. They carry the embodiment of the parents' creativity and this idea is interrupted by the possibility of passing on the 'bad gene'. It is at odds with the idea of giving the child something good. Sometimes parents feel they have harmed what is most dearly cherished and this triggers feelings of personal responsibility, blame and destructiveness.

Loss

Loss is inevitable in genetic counselling. Making a decision and resolving conflict involves a loss of an option. Knowing, whatever the implications, involves a loss of the innocence; not knowing, deprives the individual of the possibility of making use of the information personally, or for the benefit of others. There may be positive losses such as the loss of anxiety and obvious relief from worry at not having a genetic disorder. Paradoxically, not everyone feels relief at being free of the problem gene as some individuals experience the guilt of being a survivor (Tibben et al., 1990). In addition, not having the gene can interfere with the sense of belonging to the family leaving the individual isolated in wellness. Confirming the presence of a genetic disorder invariably ushers in many changes with grief or sadness being the principal emotion. The individual has to give up any idea of being invincible or immune from disease and face personal vulnerability. The knowledge of the presence of the gene invokes changes and one would be a change of identity where the earlier ideas of a healthy self-identity have to be relinquished.

Whereas everyone knows there is no such thing as perfection, having a genetic disorder can be construed by some more vulnerable personalities as an 'imperfection', or a flaw. Such ideas can trigger feelings of shame and personal dislike. Irrespective of the result, the individual will have to adjust to the new information, 'incorporate' it and own it. This involves a psychological experience of adjustment. Looking in a mirror the individual will see the same physical image, but the mental image has changed as a consequence of having personal genetic knowledge. The new internal image has to be acknowledged and will require a rewriting of the personal narrative.

When an individual discovers the presence of a genetic disorder it will have far reaching effects for others as if a stone has been thrown into a pond creating a ripple affect. It will have implications for the present children and those not yet born. It will also extend to involve the wider family with implications for siblings. In addition, relationships with a partner may be affected and, depending on how the individual adapts, friendships may be affected.

Where the change involves fertility potential, with either the impossibility of having a child or a decision not to reproduce, the loss of producing a child may take some time to resolve. Where a child has been affected by a genetic disorder or a chromosome change, the parents are faced not only with the particular problem of the disorder, but also with a disappointment. The disappointment is not directly related to the child's disorder, but more to the difference between the idealised dreamed-of child in the parents' mind and the actual child. The degree of flexibility and adjustment potential in the parents is the important factor in determining the outcome. Some families find minor problems unacceptable, whilst others find their way through major problems. There is a possibility of problems arising in the parent–child relationship which can interfere with the child-rearing practices and distort child development.

A family with a genetic history usually regard it as a responsibility to pass on that information to the next generation. The story will contain the family's view of the relevant information, the degree of disappointment fear or other emotions and the way of handling them. The story becomes part of the fabric of the family. This information falls under the category of what Carter and McGoldrick (1989) call trans-generational stress, which, as Street (1994) explains, includes patterns of relating and functioning which are transmitted down the generations (Bowen, 1978). It involves the family taboos, attitudes and expectations. There may be no family history, as for instance when carrier status is discovered with the birth of an affected child. Under that circumstance the information is new, the family as a whole is challenged and has to negotiate its way through two transitions. One relates to a birth which is a natural change in the family life cycle; the other to the adjustment the family needs to make to the affected child.

Frustration

Having a genetic disorder may seriously interfere and frustrate long-standing plans, ideas, ambitions or even ordinary living when the condition is debilitating. The individual may have to review future plans of job prospects, possible marriage or having children. It may also prevent an individual being able to have personal insurance. Varying degrees of adjustment will be necessary for the individual to live a life which includes the consequences of the genetic disorder. From the point of view of psychological management, the principal task is the resolution of anxiety and grief. For simplicity in further discussions about stress and emotions, frustration will be seen as a corollary.

Individual perception of the stress of genetic counselling

It has already been stated that although there is a potential for stress in addressing a genetic problem, the individual's appraisal will determine how it is perceived and whether it is construed as stressful. McConkie-Rosell and Sullivan (1999) have adapted Lazarus and Folkman's Theory of Stress and Coping (1984) for genetic counselling and consider that the factors influencing perception in the primary appraisal of genetic counselling are environmental, personal and social. The environmental factors refer to the disease, the severity of the disorder, availability of treatment, number of affected individuals in the family and the amount of contact with affected or carrier family members. The individual's personal experience of these facts is an important factor in establishing their meaning. The personal and social variables include self-concept, comprehensive family characteristics, the amount of social support and desire for children or grandchildren. The interaction between the environmental and personal factors is important and results in the individual experiencing varying degrees of anxiety. This is the principle determining factor in the assessment of the challenge, colouring the issue and rendering it possible or impossible. It is interesting to note that not only does anxiety influence perception, but it is also affected by perception. An anxious person will perceive a situation as difficult. Equally, perceiving a situation as difficult is anxiety provoking. A situation which is viewed as difficult, but manageable, or that has to be managed, will be approached with resolve and belief that somehow the individual will be able to cope. Conversely, a situation which is viewed as disastrous and unmanageable will trigger anxiety and result in the situation being managed defensively, or result in the emergence of symptoms. The counsellor will be familiar with these differences in everyday clinical practice. Some individuals manage to approach genetic counselling and contain their distress; other more anxious individuals avoid the issue or approach with a strong defence such as intellectualisation, or present with varying degrees of emotional disturbance.

Perception is also influenced by the previous experiences of similar issues and results in the past affecting how the present is perceived. This is particularly relevant in genetic counselling where having a test for a disorder, when other members of the family have been severely affected, will be extremely challenging. Confronting genetic issues in the present will trigger memories of past experience of illness in the family and force them to the forefront of the individual's mind. This brings alive the pain suffered as a result of the illness and includes the effect that it had on relationships.

This theoretical explanation helps the counsellor understand the important factors contributing to an individual's stress response and will direct the counselling interventions to helping the individual control anxiety.

As a result of the primary appraisal the situation will be considered stressful or not. Where the appraisal is that the situation is not stressful, it may be relatively easy to proceed with genetic counselling. When the process is perceived as a stress, a secondary appraisal is necessary and involves an analysis of coping resources.

The concept of individual appraisal and perception of stress can be represented diagrammatically (Fig. 2.1) as follows.

Coping

When faced with a challenge which is considered to be stressful, the individual has to find ways of coping to deal with the problem and reduce, or tolerate, the internal and external demands created by the stressful situation

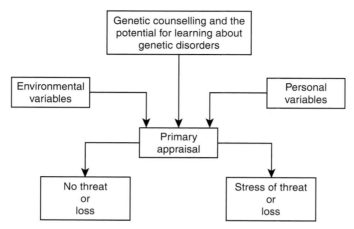

Figure 2.1   This is a simplified version of the adaptation of McConkie-Rosell and Sullivan (1999) of Lazarus and Folkman's Theory of Stress and Coping (1984).

(Folkman and Lazarus, 1985). As in the initial appraisal, coping is dependent on the environmental, personal and social factors. It draws on physical, social and psychological resources. Coping is defined as being independent of the outcome of success or failure and has two main functions: the regulation of emotions and the management of the problem. Both emotional and cognitive processing are used in most situations. The former is used to process and contain the distressing emotions; the latter includes conscious strategies of analysing the situation and acting appropriately to master the challenge, problem solve and make decisions (Cohen and Lazarus, 1979). The two are intertwined and inter-related as the effectiveness of the problem-solving depends largely on the success of the emotion-focused efforts (Easterbrook, 1959). The individual thoughts include, 'How do I see this problem?' 'What can I do to resolve it?' and 'How do I deal with the feelings it triggers?'

Folkman (1984) emphasised the importance of having control over emotions. This applies more to the negative emotions of threat and anxiety as they interfere more than positive emotions in problem-solving. In practice this means having control over the level of anxiety which, as was seen in the primary appraisal, is a key determinant in the 'stress and coping equation'.

In a genetic challenge the problem-focused coping will determine what the individual believes can be done to deal with the challenge and, in particular, whether testing and having knowledge will be of use. Berkenstadt et al. (1999) considered the individual's level of knowledge about their genetic condition gave a degree of control and helped in the problem-focused coping. McConkie-Rosell and Sullivan (1999) considered that genetic counselling interventions should be directed to reducing anxiety and enhancing control as those interventions facilitate a sense of mastery and provide an increased understanding. Other authors have described the adaptive coping strategies in response to genetic testing as hope, learning new knowledge, developing new coping methods, increased control and minimisation (Kessler, 1984; Shiloh et al., 1997).

Different coping responses

In their analysis of stress and genetic testing for disease risk Baum et al. (1997) explored the relationship between the disease and the individual's coping. They considered that the extent to which genetic testing for disease causes significant distress varies as a function of the following factors: the test results, the characteristics of the disease, the uncertainty remaining after testing, the degree of uncertainty reduction, the availability of active coping option and personal factors such as social support, optimism, perceived risk and beliefs about disease and disability. As a consequence, the interaction of all these factors results in a range of coping responses which have been described in varying ways. These include adaptive or maladaptive (McConkie-Rosell and Sullivan, 1999), or resilient, normal stress and pathological stress response (Horowitz et al., 2001). However, in this text the terminology adopted by Tibben (1993) is used – that of mature, defensive and symptomatic. In essence these differences relate to the individual management of anxiety. Grief takes a different path and will be discussed later.

It is important to realise that in some instances in genetic counselling the situation is appraised and re-appraised several times, with a series of decisions needing to be made as the consultation proceeds. In cancer genetics, prenatal testing and Huntington's disease the decision-making process is staged. It begins with the decision to ask for a consultation, is followed by a decision to be tested and have genetic information and, in many instances, a further decision is necessary. The latter may involve monitoring in cancer genetics; a decision about a pregnancy after prenatal testing; and telling the family of the genetic situation in Huntington's disease.

The mature approach

The classification of a mature approach is used when the individual recognises and acknowledges that there is a potential problem, manages the anxiety and assesses the situation without distorting reality too much. In practice, this means that an individual acknowledges the genetic problem and embarks on the counselling process with appropriate anxiety which is used to do what Janis (1958) called the 'worry work of internal mental rehearsal'. In counselling for Huntington's disease this involves the individual imagining different scenarios of having positive and negative test results. These imaginary scenes are entered into to help the individual explore the varying emotional experiences which would result. Whilst practising these scenes the individual will also be digesting the information provided. This thoughtful and responsible approach of mentally facing the dilemma, acting appropriately and learning about the disorder is a forerunner and a mental rehearsal for the actual experience of having a test result. A further factor in the successful negotiation of the difficulties in genetic counselling is the ability of individuals with a mature approach to have and use an external support system of friends and family (Rowland, 1990; Tibben, 1993).

In his research study of Huntington's disease, Tibben (1993) identifies the mature approach as one where there is some worry work and anticipation. He quotes the following examples 'I talk and read a lot about the things that could happen to me after disclosure of the results' and 'If I prove to be a gene-carrier, then I'll tell some specific friends I can trust'. In both these statements there are anticipatory fear and rehearsal and the idea of support being available and used. This way of managing the anxiety by containment and preventing it escalating, enables the individual to approach genetic counselling and manage the subsequent test result. The ability stems from an internal strength which is a result of good secure early attachment experiences (this will be elaborated in the next chapter).

The individual is likely to have had previous experience of coping with difficult and stressful situations. As a result, an internal bank of confidence builds up and acts as a reference body which can be drawn on. Each time a difficult situation is managed it adds to the internal strength and reinforces the possibility that the future can be managed, even if painful. Pursuing hope, learning information, constructing meaning, acquiring new knowledge, developing new coping methods, increasing control and minimisation have been described as constructive coping behaviours (Kessler, 1984; Shiloh et al., 1997).

The defensive approach

Individuals in this group do not have the same internal, or possibly external, resources as those who have a 'mature' approach. The situation can be improved by increasing the external support by involving more people (and that is one function of the counsellor). In addition, the individual also unconsciously affects a change internally by using mental mechanisms of defence. These help the individual cope and restore the sense of internal equilibrium.

Mental mechanisms of defence

Mental mechanisms of defence act by distorting reality, changing it in the individual's mind and so protecting the individual from being overwhelmed by anxiety. Some distortion of reality is almost inevitable, especially imme- diately after shock, when the function is to protect the individual by giving time to adjust. The defences can be useful if used appropriately and for short periods of time. They become pathological, or unhelpful, if used inappro- priately or for too long, as the distortion they effect can prevent the problem from being realistically addressed. To be constructive, the mental mech- anisms need to change with time and as the distortions lessen they allow more of reality to penetrate. The nature of the defence mechanism and the extent to which it is used will vary, with some being more helpful and mature than others. There is a wide range of different defence mechanisms which include denial of a problem, repression, rationalisation, displacement activity, intellectualising, sublimation, reaction formation and projection.

The most primitive of defences is *denial*. It is normal if used in childhood play when pretending to be someone else, but abnormal in adulthood, if used other than for a short time. It is a defence which has to be resorted to when the repertoire of defences is not very rich. It can be considered to be normal if, for example, it is used for a short time after a shock, as for instance in bereavement or after receiving bad news, but becomes abnormal if its use is prolonged. The genetic counsellor will have experience of this defence being used constructively after a test result and seeing how it changes slowly as the individual adapts to the news. The defence is less useful when it results in an individual avoiding a situation which either needs addressing, especially if it could be beneficial. For example, an individual may have a family history of cancer, yet refuse to address the difficulty and be tested for the gene. As a consequence, the individual is unable to benefit from monitoring and early detection of the disorder. The defence and avoidance is then a false protection, denying the individual the opportunity of potentially helpful knowledge. In a disorder such Huntington's disease the defence can serve different functions at different times. It is unhelpful if it prevents the individual planning or informing children. However, later on it can become constructive as it allows the individual to deny the problem and continue living a full life, instead of being preoccupied with the disorder and waiting for symptoms to appear.

Shiloh (1996) does not use the concept of mental mechanisms of defence, but has ideas which are very similar for example using the term 'defensive avoidance' to describe denial. Genetic decisions are considered to be high-stress situations and can result in two sub-optimal patterns of responsive behaviour: 'defensive avoidance' and 'hypervigilance'. The former arises when there is high conflict and pessimism about finding a good solution and testing is likely to be avoided. The latter situation arises when there is high emotionality and vacillation with a tendency to catastrophise even simple situations, with panic never far away. The situation becomes a crisis and extremely difficult to resolve.

Repression is an essential mechanism of defence. A considerable amount of life's experiences are repressed and hidden away in the unconscious, especially if the experiences are too painful to remain in the conscious mind. It would be impossible to hold all memories in the conscious mind, but equally, erasing all memories with a sweeping repression leads to enormous difficulties of not learning from experience. These 'forgotten' experiences are not readily available to the conscious mind, but dreams, slips of the tongue and humour can give tell-tale clues. However, these past memories can be retrieved from the unconscious if triggered by a similar experience in the present. For example, the painful experience of being a child in a family where a parent has suffered from Huntington's disease, may have been repressed, but the memory can be resurrected when the child becomes an adult and requests testing. The testing is then acting as a trigger releasing the memories. The counsellor needs to be alerted to the fact that a review of the family history in the counselling process can be traumatic, as it takes the individual back in time, bringing the past alive in the present. However, this 'remembering' can be helpful as it allows what could not be managed in childhood to be viewed through the more capable eyes of an adult. Anxiety provoking experiences of childhood can be revisited and worked through in adulthood, especially if helped by a counsellor.

The defence of *rationalisation* involves making plausible and more acceptable explanations to hide the real story or feeling. It changes something unpleasant into a more pleasant alternative. For example, a person who has a family history of a genetic problem may choose not to be tested, rationalising that there is nothing much that can be done to change the situation, so there is no point in knowing. In another example, a person who is unable to have children may rationalise and turn the situation round by denying any desire to have children.

Displacement is the defence used when an emotion is transferred from the relevant event or a person onto someone or something else. For example, instead of facing the anger felt towards a partner for having a particular gene, the emotion is displaced and expressed as being angry with a partner for a minor irritation, or with someone else. Alternatively, in *displacement activity* an individual may become very active cleaning the house after an upset, so making a displaced attempt to symbolically clean away the unpleasant emotions.

The desire to learn more about the problem, to understand and gain more information is constructive use of *intellectualisation*. However, if used excessively, then it can become an intellectual defence which protects the individual from facing the emotional pain. Most counsellors will have experience of people who want more and more details and spend a considerable amount of energy searching for answers. The danger is that too much intellectualisation separates ideas from emotions and leaves the emotions unrecognised and unprocessed.

With the defence of *sublimation*, unacceptable feelings are channelled into more socially acceptable activities. For example, a parent, who has a child with a serious disability, may become very committed to a support group and this 'good' activity helps alleviate the distress or 'bad' feelings. Sublimation is constructive and certainly creates something useful, but hopefully not at the expense of recognising the distress.

Reaction formation is a defence which turns an emotion upside down and, instead of experiencing a negative emotion, the individual expresses the more positive opposite. An example would be of a mother who finds her anger with her handicapped child so unacceptable that, unconsciously, she goes to abnormal lengths to please the child.

With the defence of *projection*, unpleasant feelings are not owned by the individual, but are 'pushed outside' and ascribed to others. Instead of acknowledging personal dissatisfaction with doctors, for example, the individual may speak about the fact that a neighbour was dissatisfied with a doctor in another hospital. The feeling of dissatisfaction has been personally disowned and projected into another.

Mental mechanisms of defence are very personal and can endure across different situations with a particular defensive style being characteristic of the individual. However, the style is not fixed and, in a supportive counselling relationship, the individual may be able to use a more mature approach and contain the emotions. The following examples illustrate the use of different mental mechanisms of defence.

Examples

1. In a family where the father had a history of Polycystic Kidney disease, the three adult children had been tested and all were confirmed as having the gene. However, only one makes use of routine blood pressure and metabolic monitoring. In a counselling session she described how she and her siblings think and behave differently. She explained that her brother did not want to be tested. 'What he doesn't know doesn't hurt him; my sister, she's in the middle she isn't sure. My brother is intelligent, but he keeps his head in the sand. Me, I want to know and face all the check ups'.

   Here we see three different ways of dealing with the problem and handling anxiety. The identified patient acknowledges the problem and seeks information, a brother uses denial and avoidance, whilst a sister is ambivalent and vacillates between the two.

2. In the following extract of a counselling session a young woman revealed how she vacillated, struggling to resolve her dilemma by going in and out of denial.

   The counsellor asked, 'What sort of result did you think you might get?' and she replied, 'I don't know. I haven't thought about it at all. ... after I had it done then, it just went out of my mind ... I am not worried, I am just happy to know.'

She then revealed more of her thinking, 'I just think, it might never happen, sort of thing, I just think it might never happen – hopefully, you know … If it happens, it happens, it's just not knowing. I'm not bothered. You know, I'm not worried. Well I am a worrier, but not as my mother'.

She then showed insight into the human mind, 'I keep thinking, oh it won't bother me, but if I do have it … it will bother me loads. It's different when you don't know, then you think, oh well, it wouldn't bother me'.

This extract shows a woman attempting to master anxiety by denial, yet knowing it does not work. She understands the way the human mind changes and plays with reality and that sometimes, only when reality is confirmed, is anxiety really acknowledged.

3. Defences can change over time and those used immediately after receiving bad news can change as people begin to work through their upset. The following extract of a counselling session illustrates a change over time. The patient is very reflective and has well-established thinking and language skills. These enable her to be able to describe the changes she experiences and how, in the process of adjustment, she recognises the painful reality of her situation.

Extract

P: When I was told in the clinic I had the gene, I just said, I'm not surprised, I've always known. But you know I didn't really know, I was just thinking if I think I've got it then it can't be worse and it might be better. When we left the clinic I got in the car and my husband said 'let me drive' but I said 'no I want to drive, I'm fine'. But do you know what I did? I reversed out and went bang straight into another parked car … I started to cry and just couldn't stop.

C: I guess you were very shocked when you left the clinic and your awareness was not as it usually is. Crashing into the car was another crisis which frightened you, as if you hit something else which threw you off course. So perhaps you were crying about your result and the car.

P: I was. I suddenly went into 'stop'; I felt I couldn't do anything. My husband put me to bed and I just cried and slept.

C: It sounds as if you were very shocked.

P: I felt numb when I woke up. I started to remember what had happened and thought, 'No, it isn't true'.

C: Mmmh.

P: Sometimes I would realise and at other times it was like a dream.

C: You were struggling to realise what had happened but it was too much to take in.
P: I thought I was prepared but I wasn't, you think you are but until it happens you don't really understand. And even now because I'm no different I still think it might never happen.

C: You are working quite hard to adjust to the news but it's not easy, I guess you are frightened of what it means.
P: Oh, am I frightened especially when I think of my mother and how she was and now I have to tell my kids. I've been so angry as well, 'why me' I've kept saying and 'please not my kids'. But now sometimes I accept that it's going to be like this, 'this is the situation'. It was as if I am trying to wake up out of a dream or something.

C: Exactly.

C: Almost pretending …
P: I didn't want to admit it to myself, but I think that was a normal reaction.

C: And so as time has gone by?
P: It's changed.

C: There's been a realisation to it and an adjustment, some internal adjustment.
P: There's been some; I don't say it's been fully to be honest. I'm still angry and depressed and cry but … more sad inside now.

C: Okay.
P: Because at the end of the day it is still a shock to the system … maybe sort of levelling off, slowly coming to terms with it.

This extract illustrates the struggle between denial and realisation and its resultant anger and depression, which as the individual stated, is normal. Horowitz et al. (2001) comment on the way the feelings change with time. They describe the process of responding to a test result as having a number of phases which include outcry, denial, an intrusive phase (characterised by unbidden thoughts and sudden pangs of emotion), working through and completion.

Symptomatic

Symptoms of anxiety emerge when the individual cannot manage to process or contain the emotion and the mental mechanisms of defence fail, are inappropriate for the situation, or are used for too long. Anxiety may present in its many different disguises, some of which include: overt anxiety, panic attacks, intrusive thoughts which preoccupy and dominate thinking, physical symptoms or acting out behaviour where the individual is angry or self harms.

In his analysis of defence and coping mechanisms in 20 individuals at risk of Huntington's disease. Tibben (1993) found that the level of anxiety had a greater discriminating power than the test result itself and was correlated with intrusive feelings and thoughts, strong avoidance behaviour and a decrease in the level of hopelessness. In contrast, carriers with low anxiety showed the least avoidance behaviour and the highest level of hopelessness. He also described a maladaptive pattern where there was acting out, obsessive preoccupation or attacks against the self. Horowitz et al. (2001) noted that if the response is intense or prolonged the outcome is a stress response syndrome, with symptoms which can resemble a post-traumatic stress disorder. The symptoms include intrusive thoughts, pangs of fear, irrational avoidance behaviour and impulsive decision-making. They predicted that 20% of those who receive grim news of genetic risk for a dire disorder will have a stress response. In a study of the effects of pre-symptomatic testing for Huntington's disease over a 3-year period, Tibben et al. (1997) reported there was only slight change from the baseline in intrusive thoughts and avoidance in both carriers and non-carriers. The shock or the relief of the test result was only evident after 1 week with an increase in intrusive thoughts in carriers after 6 months, before returning to the baseline at 3 years.

Figure 2.2 diagrammatically represents the relationship between primary and secondary appraisal, stress and different ways of coping.

Processing grief

So far the coping response has referred to the management of fear and anxiety. The different ways of processing of grief will now be discussed. In processing grief there is a similar pattern to that seen in the management of anxiety. Some individuals process their grief and move towards resolution; others have a prolonged experience or get stuck at a particular point. These two paths parallel the mature and defensive management of anxiety whilst in the symptomatic group individuals become very depressed. The terminology usually used to describe these different patterns with respect to grief is normal, atypical or chronic and symptomatic.

Grief is the experience of loss, a long process where the central task is the ability to say goodbye and mourn the loss. Mourning is the process that has to be gone through in adapting to the loss. The term bereavement usually is

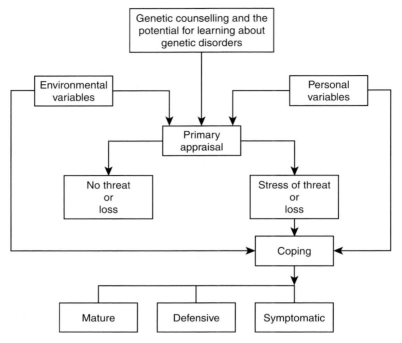

Figure 2.2   Adapted from McConkie-Rosell and Sullivan (1999) of Lazarus and Folkman's Theory of Stress and Coping (1984).

reserved for the loss of a loved one through death and is used as a template for understanding other losses. Engel (1961) considers the loss of a loved one to be as psychologically traumatic as being severely wounded physically.

The genetic counsellor will be very familiar with the grieving process as there are many different forms of loss around genetic issues. Even knowledge involves loss since it changes what was. The genetic counsellor sees people at varying points on the grief pathway as they progress from shock and denial to acceptance and adjustment. Although the loss can vary in its nature, the template for understanding the process is that of bereavement, the loss of a loved one.

In his work on bereavement, Parkes (2001) does not consider that the pathway is a series of stages to be gone through in a linear fashion, but rather describes four phases: Phase I is the period of numbness which occurs close to the time of the loss; Phase II is the period of yearning, where there is often denial of the permanence of the loss; Phase III is characterised by disorganisation and despair where ordinary functioning is a struggle and in Phase IV there is re-organisation of behaviour and a return to every day living. Worden (1991) picks up Freud's idea of grief work and describes four tasks of mourning which he considers to be of use clinically. They are: to accept the reality of the loss, to work through the pain and grief, to adjust to an environment in which the deceased is missing (which involves internal, external and spiritual adjustments) and finally to emotionally relocate the deceased and move on with life. The last task suggests that it is necessary to find a place for the deceased, recognising that there is a continuing bond which does not interfere with the development of a new life.

In a recent study, Machin and Spall (2004) propose that grief reactions fall into three broad categories: 'overwhelmed', 'balanced' and 'controlled'. Using a research tool, the Adult Attitude to Grief scale, which had been devised earlier (Machin, 2001), it was possible to map the responses of individual clients to the losses. By inviting individuals to think about themselves in this way, they suggest that the scale can also help as a clinical tool to give structure to the individual narrative of clients and to convey the significance of their loss in a way which would have a new meaning for the client. This therapeutic approach incorporates a combined Person-Centred, narrative and cognitive approach to create a renewed sense of agency and equilibrium. In practice, this means listening to the story to understand the individual's experience (Person-Centred), helping in the development of a story which is more healing (narrative) and challenging self-defeating thoughts (cognitive).

The grieving process involves a profound internal sense of loss where the individual feels sadness which can sometimes extend to depression, distress or anger. It can be experienced as being like a physical pain, or an emptiness which is occasionally described as feeling like a hole inside. It is frequently accompanied by changes in behaviour with periods of restlessness, agitation and a state of high arousal alternating with periods of withdrawal from the world. This is the outward sign of an internal searching and longing to regain the lost person. The early experience of shock, numbness and disbelief gives way to, or is punctuated by, a realisation of the loss and the sense of internal emotional pain. Sadness, anger and frustration are common and intense longing can dominate the individual's thinking. Hearing familiar sounds associated with the lost loved one, or sensing their presence, are experienced by many people.

When a loved one has been lost, those remaining will use photographs or treasured possessions to help in the psychological adaptation. The mourner goes in and out of the grieving process, moves forward towards adaptation, making headway, only then to perhaps relapse and feel the pain as if it were new. Memories of events, shared moments or relationship experiences of how things were are brought to the surface, thought about with longing and sadness, before the thoughts can be relinquished. For some people the grieving process becomes physical and active, full of rituals such as taking flowers to the grave or lighting a candle on the birthday of the dead loved one. At these times the dead are remembered, but in their absence; thus remembering the life that was and, the loss which remains.

It is always difficult to demarcate exactly the normal grieving process, but the counsellor's clinical experience will include examples of grief becoming atypical or distorted, exaggerated, prolonged or stuck at a particular point on the path. For instance, a room left as it was the day a loved one died is a sort of mummification. It suggests that the dead person cannot be let go to remain as a memory. Instead, there is a 'hanging on' in an attempt to maintain things as they were. Facing the absence can sometimes feel unbearable. One such example is of a family who left the room of their dead child untouched, leaving the bed linen unchanged to try and preserve the smell of the child. The family were trying to hold onto a living experience and literally attempting to make sure that the impression of a life remained. In another example, a mother kept a lock of her dead child's hair in a locket which she constantly wore so holding the memory, and a physical part of the child, close to her heart.

The grieving process can become symptomatic in a number of ways. It can be hampered by a defensive approach such as denial or the opposite can happen when the individual feels overwhelmed by emotions and fears fragmentation. The most common symptom of unresolved grief is depression. A certain amount of depression is normal as part of the grieving process, but if it becomes fixed or interferes with ordinary living and results in the individual withdrawing from the world, then it will require more specialist help. The counsellor will know that the grieving process can be a slow working through of feelings which can be helped by offering a supportive relationship. Such an intervention will enable the individual to adjust and reconfigure their life.

Other emotions frequently experienced in genetic counselling

Guilt and shame are emotions which are frequently felt by individuals in genetic counselling. In everyday life they are often fused and confused.

Erikson (1950) has pointed out that the confusion happens because there is a developmental tendency for shame to be submerged by guilt, as both develop as part of conscience and are experienced in the context of having done something wrong. In the psychoanalytical theory of development, conscience develops around the resolution of the oedipal complex when the boy resolves conflicts and desires and identifies with his father. In his developmental schema, Erikson separated shame by proposing that it arose at the stage of conflicts around what he calls the stage of 'Shame versus Doubt and Autonomy'. It is important to understand the origins of shame and guilt and to clarify important differences to help the counsellor make the appropriate response. As Kessler (1984) has indicated, guilt arises as a result of mechanisms within the individual, where there is a harsh internal judgement with very high standards demanded. In contrast, shame arises in the context of feeling inadequate in the eyes of the external world, the internal judgement having been projected onto others. In Archer's (1993) study of this subject he uses Chasseguet-Smirgel's (1985) clarification of these two emotions. He explained that they derive from a stage of development where there is a struggle with 'good/bad' and 'right/wrong', such that 'bad' and 'wrong' can feel equally applicable. He further quotes Chasseguet-Smirgel (1985) who differentiates the two by stating, 'whereas guilt is aroused when a limit is touched or transgressed, shame arises when a goal is not reached'. Put more simply, shame is linked to a feeling of helplessness and poor self-image, whereas guilt arises from an excessive growth of conscience. Guilt and shame, in moderation, are part of the developmental socialisation process. They become problematic when they are excessive, a situation which probably arises as a result of unsatisfactory early relationships. Those prone to feelings of guilt have possibly been exposed to a considerable degree of harshness in their early years; those who experience shame may have had a lack of support at the stage of awareness that there is an outside world where they can be judged. In both instances there appears to be an absence of self-compassion and tolerance in their adult internal world which probably reflects the lack of understanding and care in the early emotional environment. Alternatively, it may indicate how our present society is intolerant of anything other than perfection.

How then can the genetic counsellor help in assuaging guilt or shame? Logically there has been no wrong-doing, but reassurances along logical lines, or normalisation, are singularly unhelpful. Kessler (1984) rightly suggests that the feelings need to be explored and put in the context of the individual's history and psychological make-up. In addition it may be useful to consider whether excessive guilt is part of a grieving process which has become stuck and needs to be unlocked. This can be done by refocusing on any loss which has not been fully acknowledged and helping the individual move along the path of grief. Guilt can also be a cover for anger or indeed exist because of angry feelings. Alternatively, guilt is easily triggered in the 'perfectionist' and can be experienced as a punishment for some minor or major misdemeanour.

The individual's belief in shame is that a personal inadequacy or vulnerability has been exposed to the world and results in a lowering of self-esteem and stimulates a desire to hide away. The genetic disorder is experienced as an attack on the sense of self, a narcissistic injury. It occurs in vulnerable individuals who have not experienced a loving relationship which includes an acceptance of faults and imperfections. Shame is therefore more difficult to work with as it can indicate a more sensitive and vulnerable personality in need of considerable support and empathy. The vulnerability and shame are often hidden under the cloak of anger and rage at the genetic discovery, and the counsellor may find the situation quite challenging. Attempting to understand the anger is often more productive than reacting to it or logically trying to reason it away. Both guilt and shame can be helped by an empathic and compassionate relationship with a counsellor who is prepared to listen to understand the individual's make-up and explore how it is generating this particular response to a genetic problem. When working with guilt, the counsellor is attempting to moderate the patient's internal harshness, encouraging the story to be told and seen afresh without judgement. Working with shame, the counsellor's interventions are directed towards positive affirmation of areas of competence. The individual is encouraged to expose what is considered shameful where it can be seen and re-appraised in an understanding and supportive relationship.

These emotions can be felt in many different genetic situations, but most commonly they are seen in parents who have a child with genetic problems. The problem can be construed as punishment or linked inappropriately to something one of the parents has done, either during or before the pregnancy. Both the emotions call for the counsellor to understand the parents' sense of responsibility or inadequacy in a gentle supportive professional relationship, offering acceptance and compassion, which the parents cannot generate for themselves. Counsellors are in an ideal position to help at such times of a family crisis by being interested companions, exploring why the couple are giving themselves such a hard time, helping them face the disappointment to be able to let go and move on.

It is worth remembering that, if these feelings have arisen in the context of disappointment and grief, then they could be considered to be part of a 'blocked' grief process. Consequently, if the counsellor offers an understanding relationship, the individual, or couple, may be able to leave behind the punitive feelings of guilt and shame and work through their sadness.

In summary, in this chapter the emphasis has been on decision-making and coping with a test result, the two key elements in genetic counselling. They have been understood in the theoretical context of psychological stress, which gives the counsellor a framework to understand the challenge to the individual and the adjustments which have to be made. Clinical experience illustrates that there are infinite ways of coping with the psychological challenge and that individuals have their own idiosyncratic ways of managing the challenge. These will be determined by their perception of the problem, previous experiences of managing psychological stress, internal resources, as well as the immediate support network. The inter-relationship between stress and individual perception clarifies why individuals approach and experience genetic counselling in so many varied ways.

Summary points

Genetic counselling attempts to deal with uncertainty about an individual's genetic status. In giving an answer it may not remove uncertainty but rather, change it.

Genetic counselling is different from other consultations since it is about knowledge and its key elements are decision-making and coping with a result.

Genetic counselling has the potential to be psychologically stressful since it involves a change and demands an adjustment. It can trigger anxiety, grief and frustration. Stress is only experienced if the individual perceives the process as a threat, and the individual is then challenged to cope. Stress can interfere with decision-making.

Coping involves cognitive and emotionally focused processing working together to enable the individual to cope. Essentially coping involves the management of anxiety and grief.

Individuals differ in their management of anxiety and grief and frustration and fall into one of three groups; mature, defensive or symptomatic.

3

Understanding individual difference in genetic counselling using attachment theory

The last chapter clarified how individuals differ in their management of anxiety and grief and linked it to the perception of genetic counselling and whether it was seen as stressful or not. In addition, individuals were shown to differ in their coping responses and to fall broadly into one of three groups: mature, defensive and symptomatic. This is particularly relevant to the counsellor as it explains different approaches and responses to genetic counselling. There are however individual differences in a number of other areas which have relevance for genetic counselling. These differences relate to the way a genetic family story is told, the thinking behind decision-making and the nature and pattern of relationship with the counsellor. All these differences of individual behaviour can be understood by referring to the concepts contained in attachment theory. The theory provides a framework which explains how these differences have arisen and how they are played out in genetics. Armed with these concepts, the counsellor will be equipped to recognise different patterns of behaviour and relating and to connect them to underlying attachment patterns. The counsellor can then adjust their personal response correspondingly so enhancing the professional relationship.

Attachment theory

Attachment theory is an up-to-date approach now being adopted and integrated into the different theoretical bases and thinking of the various schools of psychotherapy. It was conceived in the post-Freudian era and, in recent times, there has been a resurgence of interest from researchers, psychiatrists, psychotherapists and counsellors. It arose as a reaction to what was seen as patriarchal psychoanalysis and shifted the emphasis from Freud's ideas of internal drives and conflict (his basis of understanding of the underlying motives driving the individual), to the individual's need for protection, comfort and security. This need is vital for survival in infancy, but attachment needs continue to be important throughout adult life. The change in focus, from the Freudian intrapsychic domain to the relationship between the individual and the actual environment, emphasises the importance of real interpersonal or relational links between people.

Those working in genetic counselling do not need to have a psychotherapeutic training but, they do need an understanding of themselves in relation to their patients and the way the early attachment patterns can affect the dynamic. Attachment theory is a user-friendly framework where the concepts fit well with genetic counselling and can enrich the process.

It was conceived by John Bowlby (1979) and brings together ideas from psychoanalysis, ethology and evolutionary biology. The basis of the study centres on the separation and reunion behaviour of young children from their carer and arises from the observation that children behave differently on separation. The central concepts of attachment theory include: the secure base and individual behaviour, the regulation of emotion, narrative competence, self-reflection and internal working models (Holmes, 2001). These ideas will be presented individually and their application to genetic counselling elaborated.

Secure base and individual behaviour

Attachment theory begins from the basis that we all need to interact and explore the outside world – we need to investigate and take part in the social context in which we exist. To do this it is important to have a confidence in ourselves and our ability to express ourselves effectively in the social world. This confidence begins to be formed in the first few days of an infant's life. As we are vulnerable at this time, we need to be able to feel secure, especially when under threat. Attachment theory was conceived around this need of the infant seeking proximity and comfort from the mother who provides protection, soothing and safety, especially at times of threat of separation, illness and fatigue. A secure base is formed when there is a particular quality to the early relationship between the mother and infant. The term refers to the sense of safety and security which develops from the early attachment experiences with the principal carer and, for simplicity in this text, the mother is taken to be the caregiver. The degree of security experienced by the infant forms the basis of a way of describing people and their attachment pattern.

The 'good-enough' mother (Winnicott, 1971) provides both physical and emotional care for her infant. The quality of that care is dependent on the degree of responsiveness of the mother. The ability of the mother to monitor the child's internal state and respond appropriately, determines her level of attunement to her baby. When successful, the mother's understanding provides a secure base, which is, at this early stage, both a physical and a psychological space, which the infant can trust and feel safe in. The mother's emotional attunement to the infant and her understanding of the infant's needs enable her to monitor the infant's internal state and respond appropriately. The accuracy of the mother's interpretation of the child's emotional state is a key factor. Ainsworth et al. (1978) identified attunement, sensitivity and responsiveness as relationship characteristics facilitating the development of a secure base. Sometimes the mother plays and stimulates, at other times calms as appropriate, but most importantly, she moderates the infant's discomfort and transforms it, alleviating the distress. As a consequence, the infant feels physically and emotionally assured and trusting. At this early stage the secure base has both physical and emotional elements. The infant is held physically in the mother's arms and emotionally in the mother's mind. In a similar way a counsellor monitors the emotional state and the well-being of the patient. For example, there may be times when the counsellor concludes that the patient may be too upset to listen and so delays giving further information, or gives more time supporting and helping the patient to do further emotional processing.

The mother's relationship with her developing infant changes over time and is related to the changing level of competence of the developing child. With a secure base as a place of safety, the child can confidently explore the world and personal talents. The mother supports the child's initiative and growing competence and in so doing facilitates the child learning appropriate skills. She also protects the child from physical stresses and harm and from being overwhelmed by too much anxiety. She balances knowing when to support initiative and when to protect from unseen danger. Most importantly, the mother makes sense of the child's emotions and, in an appropriate emotional tone, reflects back her understanding of the child's experience, using language and giving it a name. As a result, she soothes and converts unmanageable distress into something which can be contained and alleviated. This is the beginning of the development of an emotional language, not only between mother and child, but also within the child. With an internal language the developing child begins to think, assess and, most importantly, learns to have control over emotions. The mother's accurate interpretation is the initial external control of the child's emotional states which becomes replaced by the child learning personal internal control.

In contrast, when the mother's attunement is insufficient, or is inaccurate, the secure base is not established. An insecure attachment is then established and the difference between the two is reflected in the behaviour of the child on separation and, more generally, how emotions are regulated. A child who has experienced a secure attachment can tolerate separation and work through its accompanying anxiety and grief, whereas it is more problematic for those who have an insecure attachment pattern. Ainsworth et al.'s (1978) contribution to attachment theory was their invention of the 'strange situation'. In this experiment they observed the behaviour of young children on separation from the mother and related it to the attachment experience. This enabled a classification of secure or insecure attachment to be formulated. The securely attached child is able to tolerate the separation with moderate degrees of protest and distress, return to play and welcome the mother on her return. The insecurely attached is not as well equipped to tolerate the separation and three different patterns can be identified: avoidant, ambivalent and disorganised. In an insecure avoidant attachment pattern there is little protest on separation, the child remains focused on toys and dismisses the mother on her return remaining relatively unemotional throughout. With an ambivalent attachment pattern, the child becomes overwhelmed with distress and is not able to be consoled, clings to mother on her return and is unable to settle to play. With the third less common attachment pattern, a disorganised attachment, the infant displays considerable disturbance in the parent's presence with chaotic or unpredictable behaviour. Although it is the least common, the genetic counsellor may have experience of individuals who have a disorganised attachment pattern. For example, a child, who has been brought up by a parent who had Huntington's disease, may have been exposed to extremely disturbed behaviour and unpredictable child-rearing practices. The counsellor might suspect a disorganised attachment when an adult tells such a story in genetic counselling.

Holmes (2004) clarifies that the hypo- and hyper-activation of the attachment system in avoidant and ambivalent patterns are adaptive responses to sub-optimal care-giving. In contrast, the disorganised attachment is non-adaptive and has more striking links to psychopathology. Main's theory was that it represents an 'approach-avoidance dilemma' (Main, 1995). A frightened child will turn to an attachment figure for comfort and safety. If, however, the attachment figure is also a source of threat, the child is paralysed not knowing which way to turn.

The two main forms of insecure attachment patterns can be thought of as polar opposites in terms of the management of emotions; in the avoidant pattern, emotions are denied or minimised in an attempt to contain or control, whilst in the ambivalent pattern the emotions are heightened and poured out. In the less common disorganised pattern, there is considerable unpredictability in behaviour and emotions.

The determining factor governing the nature of attachment a mother establishes with her infant will be the mother's management of her own negative emotional experiences. Defensiveness in the mother may lead to a lack of understanding or dismissal of the infant's anxiety, creating an avoidant attachment for the infant. Alternatively, the mother's incomplete understanding of her infant's states induces a preoccupation with anxiety and an ambivalent attachment pattern. Conversely, a mother who can accept and process her own negative emotions is able to tolerate and moderate her infant's emotional experiences and offer herself as a secure attachment figure. As a consequence, the mother's understanding and love gives the child the experience of being able to process emotions and manage personal distress.

Research has pointed to the predictive power of attachment status in infancy for subsequent behaviour with a correlation between the attachment pattern at 1 year and at school entry (Bretherton, 1991). However, the secure or insecure attachment patterns, established early in life, are not fixed in tablets of stone. The insecure attachment patterns can change if the growing child or adult is afforded an emotionally supportive and more attuned relationship (Howes, 1999). Attachment theory is not directly developmental, but White (2004) refers to Harwood et al. (1995) who explain that the early foundations initiate developmental trends and these make achievement of later optimal functioning more or less difficult. In this way early attachment patterns are either assets, or handicaps, interacting with later life circumstances.

In adults the secure base may take the form of an external figure, a partner or other members of the present family or friends who become important at times of stress. However, in adults it is important to realise that the secure base is principally a representation of security within the individual psyche. It is an attachment state of mind and has been developed as an adaptation to early experiences. Main and Goldwyn (1995) devised the Adult Attachment Interview (AAI) which is a semi-structured psychodynamic assessment session which focuses on the form and structure of the individual's narrative. Detailed questions are asked about relationships with parents and others with particular emphasis on losses and separations to include how the individual coped with them. It enables a classification into secure-autonomous, insecure dismissive, insecure preoccupied, and disorganised or unresolved. Holmes (2001) has used this description of how a secure early attachment is revealed in adult life 'by the ways people talk about their lives, their past and in particular their relationships and associated pain', and described it as narrative competence. It is an expression of a representation in adulthood of an early experience.

Regulation of emotions

The ability to deal with separation, the hallmark of a secure attachment pattern, is an indicator that the anxiety of separation and the sadness of loss can be managed and that other challenges can be dealt with. The experience of repeated success in managing difficulties builds up an internal strength and self-belief, which can be used as an internal reference in the future.

In contrast, an insecure attachment handicaps the individual in containing anxiety and regulating the emotional experience of challenging situations. As a result, in keeping with their attachment pattern, the individual either uses a minimising style, dismissing the significance of a situation and any emotions, or perceives it is as a catastrophe, displaying a considerable amount of emotion which is not easily settled.

In addition, the securely attached individual is likely to have meaningful relationships in the present and be able to enlist help at difficult times from supportive friends and family – as a consequence drawing on support from inside and, outside of themselves.

Applying the understanding of the secure base and regulation of emotions to genetic counselling, it becomes clear that the different ways individuals approach and response to genetic counselling are related to individual attachment patterns and the ease or difficulty in managing anxiety and grief. With a secure attachment pattern, an individual would be able to approach genetic counselling with appropriate anxiety, confront the reality of possibly having a genetic disorder, analyse the situation, request a consultation and contain the anxiety generated. Further, following a result, the anxiety will be contained and grief processed, demonstrating the possession of a flexible repertoire of cognitive or emotional processing skills. The feelings can therefore be felt, recognised, contained or processed and not interfere with appropriate action. This is equivalent to the mature classification of anxiety management referred to in the previous chapter. In contrast, with an insecure pattern a more defensive approach and reaction will be result, ranging from dismissal to extreme distress. Thus the mature, defensive and symptomatic classification of anxiety described in the last chapter, can now be understood as reflecting different early attachment patterns and management of emotions.

In addition, the individual attachment style is reflected in the professional relationship. A securely attached person is able to set up a relationship with relative ease and discuss the issues with the appropriate emotions being expressed. In contrast, in order to establish a working relationship with the individual who has an insecure attachment pattern, the counsellor will need to be very attentive and adjust their own style. The patient with a dismissive pattern may appear distant and cautious and will need the counsellor to respect the style and to give time to allow the patient to 'warm up'. The counsellor can then make an attempt to gently introduce the anxiety provoking elements which have been dismissed. The patient with a preoccupied pattern will need the counsellor's help to contain emotions and keep the focus as the heightened emotions can at times dominate. When there is a disorganised attachment, the counsellor will need to adjust to changing approaches and unpredictability. It is difficult to predict how individuals with a disorganised pattern will respond to genetic counselling.

In order to relate to these different styles, the counsellor can use the mother's way of attuning to her infant as a model. The counsellor, like the good-enough mother, will be monitoring the patient's emotional state and know when to challenge, stimulate, sooth or calm a situation. In so doing, the counsellor is attempting to balance the insecure attachment and provide the missing element, or to create a greater sense of security so the patient will be freer to think and feel.

It is also important for the counsellor to be aware of their own attachment state of mind, as it will influence the degree of emotional availability which can be used in the professional relationship. Dozier et al. (1994) found that insecure clinicians tended to reinforce their clients insecure attachment styles, whereas secure clinicians were able to offer an opportunity to redress the difficulties.

In this way, by focusing on the professional relationship and the degree of attunement, the consultation space is being reframed as a potentially secure-enough base for the patient to work on the psychologically difficult issues triggered in genetic counselling. Genetic counselling cannot change attachment states of mind on a permanent basis but, by providing an attuned relationship, the counsellor may be able to create an experience which allows the individual to explore different ways of thinking and feeling which are more conducive to decision-making.

Narrative competence

In attachment theory the emphasis is on how the story is told and alerts the counsellor to listen for more than the content of the story. In particular, it includes an assessment of changes in voice, contradictions, discrepancies, gaps, hesitancies, etc. Holmes (1996) has placed considerable emphasis on the importance of this story telling ability and has called it, narrative competence. The linguistic style of the story of a securely attached person (autonomous) is one which is told in the first person, neither dismissively nor allowing emotions to overwhelm, valuing attachments and punctuating the narrative with the appropriate degree of emotionality. The storyteller reveals that pain and discomfort can be managed and involves the listener by clarifying the meaning and making sure that the story makes sense and is understood.

Insecurely attached individuals with a dismissive pattern are not coherent and will have poor recall, denigrate attachments and their meaning and tell an impoverished story. The story of those with an overtly anxious preoccupied pattern will take a rambling discourse, where there is a preoccupation with the past and the emotions are high, held onto and at times overwhelm. That of an individual with a disorganised pattern will show lapses and inconsistencies or sudden changes and punctuated with unpredictable outbursts of upset.

The individual's narrative is particularly important in genetic counselling as it contains an individual's story of the history of the gene across the generations. The degree of narrative competence will reveal not only the attachment state of mind, but also factual misconceptions and the idiosyncratic meaning given to the genetic family history. The family mythology which has been transmitted across the generations may be at odds with the scientific story of the gene. The discrepancy between the two stories will involve the counsellor in varying degrees of psychological work to ensure that the genetic information is understood. The securely attached individual will be able to make the appropriate adjustments, let go of past ideas and take in new information to develop a more accurate story. That process will be more difficult for those with an insecure attachment. Those with an insecure dismissive pattern will possibly minimise the significance of the genetic information, or deal with it in an emotionally detached manner: whereas those with a preoccupied style will be overwhelmed by emotions so that the information may not be heard correctly or will be exaggerated in its significance. It may be helpful for the counsellor to consider balancing the individual's attachment style and his/her characteristic way of handling emotions. This would lead the counsellor to use complementary facial expressions; remaining serious when the individual is light-hearted or dismissive and looking thoughtfully doubting when the individual is exaggerating.

Self-reflection and thinking processes

Attachment theory gives an understanding of an important way of thinking, referred to as reflective functioning, which Fonagy (1994) relates to an early secure attachment experience. He considers it to be the basis of the theory of mind, or mentalisation and to be at the core of self-structure. It is the ability to think about oneself in the third person, as if stepping back from oneself to observe. It enables a person to understand their own behaviour, to experience, observe and reflect, and also to understand that others have feelings too. It enables an individual to understand another's mind and underpins the ability to be intimate and to consider how another is feeling.

A story told with self-reflection would include memories of early relationships and events which would be told with a quality of integration and openness. It would convey an impression that early experiences had been thought about and dealt with. The ability to self-reflect also plays a very important part in helping the individual control emotions. Instead of being overwhelmed, the individual can think about being upset and so process and regulate the emotional state. This ability to experience and to think about an emotional state begins in childhood with the mother thinking for the child and conveying that by understanding, empathising. In that way the mother makes sense of the child's experience. It was explained earlier that, with ongoing development, this experience is internalised and built-up to give the growing child confidence in the ability to process difficult experiences. The insecurely attached adult has not had this experience in infancy to the same degree and will be limited by a restricted ability to think about an emotional state, or consider a situation thoughtfully and so has to resort to the defensive patterns.

The ability to think in a self-reflective way is vital to the individual in their assessment and decisions-making in the genetic counselling process. It enables the individual to stand back and consider the bigger picture with balance and equilibrium and to think and feel without being dismissive or overwhelmed by the emotions.

Internal working models

Bowlby (1973) selected the term 'internal working model' to describe the individual's internal belief system which contains an internal representation of the world, attachment figures, the self and relationship patterns. It has been built up through a process of internalisation of early life experiences and directs and informs present attitudes and expectations and influences future action. As a result of being sensitively responded to, the individual with a secure attachment pattern will have a trusting approach and a belief that help is at hand to negotiate the difficulty. In contrast, where there is an insecure attachment pattern the individual will be less trusting and expect the world to be unresponsive, rejecting or dismissive.

In genetic counselling it can be seen that where there is a secure attachment pattern, the individual will approach the dilemma with optimism, believing that the situation can be managed and family and friends will help. With an insecure pattern the situation will be seen as more pessimistic with doubts about the possibility or effectiveness of help.

Application of attachment theory to genetic counselling

1. It gives a framework for the counsellor to understand how people behave differently in their perception, approach and response to genetic counselling and that the differences relate to the management of anxiety and grief and early attachment patterns.

2. It allows the consultation space to be reformulated as a potentially safe place for the patient and reframes the task of the counsellor as providing a secure-enough relationship by being an emotionally available, responsive companion. Within this space, the individual can begin to think about the meaning of genetic information and make appropriate decisions.

3. It clarifies how the counsellor has to adjust the style of relating to the individual's attachment state of mind in order to counter the patterns which are proving to be unhelpful to the patient. In general the counsellor will need to help an individual with a dismissive pattern acknowledge a situation which is being avoided and feel what is being denied. However, it requires care as more reality or emotion may be frightening and result in more dismissal. Where the individual has a preoccupied pattern with an excess of emotion and rambling discourse, the counsellor will be attempting to contain the emotions and keep the focus. Again the counsellor has to be careful as these sensitive individuals can easily feel rejected.

4. It highlights the ability to remember and tell a personal story with appropriate emotionality and thought. It also provides a framework for understanding and helping the way the story is told. The counsellor is in a position to help by either expanding, or containing the degree of emotionality, to help the individual achieve a meaningful and coherent story and prepare for the adjustments needed in a genetic consultation.

5. It places the ability to self-reflect and consider a situation thoughtfully as a mark of maturity and links this to the ability to process emotions. This thinking ability facilitates the decision-making process which is central to the counselling. By providing a secure-enough relationship to facilitate the processing of emotions the counsellor can help the individual become more reflective.

6. The provision of a secure-enough relationship by the counsellor enables an individual to be in a state of mind which can take in new information. This is important in understanding genetic inheritance and personal test results.

7. It alerts the counsellor to explore and take note of their own attachment style and how that might affect the professional relationship.

The following examples are illustrations of how thinking about attachment patterns is useful in genetic counselling.

1. The importance of early attachment pattern and the effect of an early disruption being exposed in genetic counselling

A woman requested predictive testing as her father had Huntington's disease. She was accompanied by her husband and they explained that they were worried that their son who, as a late teenager, might need to know whether there was a possibility of him carrying the Huntington's gene mutation. To date, he knew nothing of his mother's family history and they believed that he would only need to know if his mother tested positive. The woman went through the stages of the Huntington's disease protocol openly and thoughtfully and she seemed well prepared to take the test. There were no worries about how she would cope with the result. Unfortunately, she was found to have the Huntington's disease mutation and, after receiving the test result, she became extremely disturbed. She was unable to go to work, cried incessantly and was frightened to be left alone. The situation did not improve with the supportive help of a genetic counsellor and a psychiatric assessment was requested. Examination of her mental state revealed that she was clinically depressed with accompanying high anxiety which at times rose to panic at the thought of being left alone.

She improved with antidepressant medication and supportive counselling. In that counselling, the focus of her distress was on the unfairness of her test result and the story of her early relationship life. The family history took on a new relevance as she expanded her story in the counselling sessions. The facts had already been established in the early interviews before testing but, perhaps, the personal significance had not been expressed or realised. The woman tearfully explained that her mother had left the family without saying goodbye and from the age of 10 years, she and her sister had been brought up by their father who, as he became more affected by Huntington's disease, treated them both violently and unpredictably. She had been told about her mother's departure by her older sister, who had received letters from her mother. The woman repeatedly cried that she would never understand how her mother could leave in such a way and why had she never contacted her.

Her older sister had attended a genetic clinic in another part of the country, had been tested and had a good result. The patient was surprised at her sister's result as she expected her to carry the mutation. Her reasoning was that her sister had a serious drink problem and sometimes got into a very disordered state and so, in the patient's mind, it followed that her sister would have the Huntington's disease gene. Further, the woman believed that because personally she had had a more traumatic time as a child and worked hard as an adult, she would not have inherited the gene. In addition, she had found a husband who cared for her and she felt she deserved to have some goodness in her life. She was convinced that she would have the good result. This firmly held belief system had been shattered when she received her result and she changed from feeling 'together' into feeling she was 'falling apart' and could not manage. She became very reliant on her husband, needing to be close to him when she could feel safe, but could not allow him to leave her.

The counselling sessions were extremely difficult as the woman was in an almost constant state of panic. The high distress and need for the counsellor to respond to her panic was challenging. Sometimes the woman would telephone in a panic and the counsellor found it difficult to maintain an understanding approach whilst maintaining reasonable boundaries. The counsellor invited the woman to explore the panic and the idea that she had to be responded to immediately. The woman found that she could wait and, to her surprise, the urgency dissipated – she could tolerate her distress. She discovered ways of talking about her early years without being overwhelmed by upset. She began to put together how the loss of her mother had left her carrying unresolved distress for many years and deskilled her in her management of upsetting challenges. In the counselling sessions she learnt to grieve both for her present and past losses and found she could be calmer. Her depression and panic had been replaced by appropriate sadness.

This woman's traumatic early experiences of separation from her mother, and the unsatisfactory relationship with her father with his unpredictability, probably afforded her a disorganised attachment pattern. As a child she was left without a supportive adult and was not able to make sense of events or manage her anxiety and grief. In the protocol for Huntington's disease she had not shown any signs a disorganised attachment with the extremes of emotion which were seen after the test result. This suggests that she had an insecure attachment pattern which was mixed. At times it was at the dismissive end of the spectrum and at other times it swung to the preoccupied end or, alternatively, revealed a disorganised pattern with an excess of distress which could not be managed.

Her relationship with her husband and the counsellor was one of needing to stay close, clinging and demanding as she struggled with mounting panic. Not only was she unable to process the anxiety and grief at her result, but her earlier unresolved loss of her mother featured strongly in her thinking. The counselling sessions moved from the past to the present, attempting to contain and resolve upset belonging to both.

The story of this woman alerts counsellors to the significance of separation and makes the point of exploring the meaning of major life events, especially those concerned with early separation and loss. If in exploring the significance of a particular event in the family history no emotion is expressed, then it is wise to suspect a denial of feelings as covering unprocessed grief. The important determining factor in a child's recovery from loss of a caregiver is the quality of care given to support a child at that time (Rutter, 1987). Unfortunately, this woman was not offered support at the loss of her mother. Paradoxically, the woman's upset at her genetic test result helped her as it resulted in her having extra counselling. That enabled her to express and contain the emotions triggered by the present upset and those resurrected from the past.

2. Absence has meaning

The protocol for testing for the Huntington's gene consists of a series of counselling sessions to consider testing. Included in the initial meeting is the suggestion to bring a relative or friend as a support.

In the following example of a preliminary meeting, the patient attended unaccompanied and, with some degree of urgency, asked to be tested that day. He gave a history of being one of two brothers who had recently learned that their mother had died of Huntington's disease. His brother had previously attended with his wife and had a good result of being free of the Huntington's gene. This had unsettled him and he had decided he needed to know whether, like his mother, he had the Huntington's disease gene. His motivation was that he had adult children and he was worried they might want children. He described how since he had known of his brother's result, he had been plagued by the thought that he must have it, as he could not believe that both he and his brother would both be free. As a result, in the last 48 hours his panic had risen and he had thought he needed to be tested immediately to try and settle his thoughts.

The interview was dominated by the man's anxiety and the request to let him have the test that day, as he did not want to think about it too much. Knowing that he was married, the counsellor commented on the absence of his wife and asked how he had decided to come, what discussion he and his wife had and how they had made the decision for him to come alone. His answer was that he had not told her as she would dissuade him. He explained that he and his wife disagreed about him being tested and under no circumstance could his wife consider telling their children if he were to be affected. He was then asked what he thought about this difference of opinion between him and his wife and he replied that his wife could not face any stress and that she would become very agitated, especially in this area where the children might need to be told. He was invited to reflect on other stressful events in his life and how he and his wife had managed. The thought behind the question was that he might be able to remember a time when they had managed a difficulty together. Unfortunately, no memory was forthcoming. He became more and more depressed as he recounted his wife's paralysing anxiety and when asked how he had managed to comfort his wife or help her through difficulties, he replied that he could not.

The counsellor commented that he had quite a dilemma. He was frightened of being tested, because it would upset him and his wife and he was not sure how either of them would handle the upset; on the other hand, he was frightened of not knowing, as he felt he had a responsibility to his children and wanted to inform them. These thoughts plagued him. Sometimes he would conclude to go ahead; at other times he would decide to avoid the issue and please his wife.

He had not discussed any of his concerns with his adult children believing they were completely unaware of the family history. He maintained that position although the counsellor wondered whether it was possible, given his brother had already been tested. The counsellor also intimated that very often there was usually some awareness in the family, but that everyone protected the other by honouring the family culture of silence. He remained convinced that his adult children did not know and he could see no advantage in talking to them at this stage. As a family they did not share worries.

The counselling session seemed to go round in circles replicating the circularity of the man's thinking and each time it returned to the theme of the man wanting to be tested immediately. Finally, after being reassured that it would be wise to talk further, he agreed to a return visit, but he never did.

This man's insecure preoccupied attachment pattern is revealed in his high anxiety state, his intrusive thoughts and the circularity of his thinking. He had been unable to control his anxiety since he had heard of the cause of his mother's death. In addition, he described his wife as also having an insecure attachment pattern and so creating a difficulty for them as a couple. It is therefore not surprising that the couple had a problem of intimacy, difficulty in sharing problems and resolving difficulties. In a manner characteristic of an over-anxious preoccupied attachment pattern, his decision was to be tested immediately. The urgency suggests that he had difficulty finding a space in his mind to think and consider the problem. Sadly, neither he nor his wife had a sufficiently secure attachment experience to address the significance of the genetic family history and its impact on them and the future generations, without being overwhelmed with anxiety.

This interview was particularly distressing for the counsellor who found that even with the best of intentions and good counselling skills, it was extremely difficult to help the man settle to think and consider his position. Witnessing such conflict and seeing the hopelessness in the man, the counsellor could easily have been tempted to try and ease his distress by going along with his request and offering the test that day. However, the protocol, previous clinical experience and knowledge of the difficulties around an insecure attachment pattern protected the counsellor from responding to the request for immediate testing. There was every possibility that if he had been tested, he would have continued to be plagued by intrusive anxious thoughts, especially if he tested positively. Honouring the protocol was therefore not as simple as a refusal, but a pausing for further meetings, in the hope of establishing a secure-enough base for containment of his anxiety.

The theoretical basis of attachment theory and its clinical application makes sense of the counsellor's clinical experience of the individual differences revealed in genetic counselling. Most importantly, it explains how the mature, defensive and symptomatic responses to genetic counselling, which were described in the last chapter, can be understood in the context of attachment patterns. The responses can therefore be seen as a reflection of secure and insecure patterns. Understanding the link to attachment patterns allows the counsellor to respond more effectively by deciding what adjustments have to be made to establish a secure-enough base for reflection and processing of emotions.

Summary points

The key points in attachment theory are: secure base, the regulation of emotions, narrative competence, self-reflection and an internal working model.

Attachment theory fits well with the processes involved in genetic counselling and provides a framework for understanding patients and their different ways of dealing with emotions, the way they tell their story, think about themselves and their dilemma, their expectations and the nature of the relationships they establish with the counsellor.

The framework enables the counsellor to understand their own attachment pattern and how, with attunement, it is possible to establish a secure-enough base to facilitate the genetic counselling process.

4

The role and skills of the counsellor and ideas from psychotherapy

The role of the counsellor

In the genetic counselling world there is debate about the main role of the counsellor, some viewing it as providing information (Antley, 1979), whilst others emphasise the facilitation of decision-making (Hsai, 1979). Shiloh (1996) comments that in reality, willingly or not, most counsellors become decision-making counsellors. Soldan et al. (2000) are of a similar mindset and consider that in predictive testing the main aims of the interview are to assist in decision-making and to help in the preparation for a result. They differentiate between the role sometimes demanded by the system of assessing the suitability for testing and the patient-focused role of assisting in their decision-making. Horowitz et al. (2001) consider that there are two major tasks in genetic counselling: 'shock mastery', with the appraisal of the meaning of a test result and a review of the question, 'Why me?' The counsellor's role would be to facilitate the two tasks.

At first sight, the two roles of information-giver and facilitator appear to be at odds with one another. However in practice, the tension between the two roles and their different elements is not that great. The two elements may involve separate themes and processes but they are intimately linked and there is a natural follow-on process from the one to the other. The patient is given information and its meaning triggers an emotional response. If the counsellor is in tune with the patient the counsellor responsively changes from an information-giver to a facilitator. The role of the counsellor is dictated by the task of the patient. Any attempt to keep the role of the counsellor solely to being an informer is likely to fail as so much of the genetic consultation is psychological. It involves reviewing the family history, considering present and past relationships and attitudes, self-reflection, decision-making and coping. These elements have been explained in earlier chapters and the importance of processing emotions and containing anxiety has been emphasised. The theories of stress and attachment have been used to explain the psychological processes and the importance of the counselling relationship in determining the outcome. However there are additional ideas, taken from the general theory of psychotherapy, which can further inform the counsellor and help to expand the skills repertoire.

Principles from psychotherapy

The following discussion begins with the key components of the counsellor's skills repertoire which include an understanding of the structure of the interview and the elements of a therapeutic professional relationship. It is important to highlight that these skills are not specific to the role of facilitator, as they are equally important for the information-giving role. In discussing the professional relationship considerable space will be given to psychotherapeutic ideas taken from Winnicott (1971) and Bion (1959). They both emphasise the importance of the professional relationship and the attitude and skill needed for it to be helpful. In addition, they both contribute to a further understanding of the links between emotions and thinking, which are so relevant for genetic counselling.

The structure of the interview

The interview takes place within a physical space, a time space and a psychological space.

The physical space

The physical space is the concrete structure of four walls and, although the consultation may be a home visit, a clinic or even a ward setting, it is always a professional consultation and the counsellor has responsibility for how it is conducted. It is easier for the counsellor to conduct an interview on the home ground of the genetic clinic or a hospital ward than to establish a professional interview space on a visit to a patient's home, where the counsellor is a guest and on someone else's territory. Nevertheless, even on a home visit, it is still a professional consultation with the counsellor setting the scene by clarifying the purpose of the visit and finding an agreed agenda to work on.

Actually, the physical space can be anywhere, as the important interview space is an interactional space, created by the discussion which takes place between the counsellor and the individual or family. Within that space, the counsellor has responsibility for the time, focus and approach.

The time space

Time, with an attitude appropriate to an understanding relationship, creates somewhere different where the conversation is different, and people can talk about extremely painful issues. With this approach patients can bring what is relevant of their lives into the genetic counselling consultation. The interview may offer a freedom to talk meaningfully but, paradoxically, the freedom can only exist within the containment and boundary of a time limit. The function of maintaining a time frame is not simply a rigid framework which makes sure others are not kept waiting, as it is a way of containing anxiety.

A consultation can be likened to a piece of music which has a beginning, builds up in the middle and ends with a conclusion, thus giving the encounter definite shape. Using the same musical metaphor, the counsellor has the same responsibility as the conductor of an orchestra which involves holding the interview together and maybe shifting the emphasis as necessary to complete the task.

Beginning on time reflects the counsellor's level of personal organisation. It is also a mark of courtesy and respect and gives the patient the message that the counsellor recognises the importance of the interview. In contrast, if the counsellor arrives late or appears rushed it suggests to the patient that the counsellor is distracted and does not have enough space in their mind to pay attention to them. Ending on time is equally important, but can sometimes be difficult if the patient is upset when the counsellor may be persuaded to continue. It is often helpful to appreciate that the time frame is a boundary of containment and can be likened to a frame holding a picture. The boundary is another way of saying to a patient who is upset that it is possible to talk about this distressing subject, contain the emotions triggered and also come out of it. It gives the patient the experience of not being dominated by a story, or being overwhelmed by emotions and that it is possible to go in and out of an experience, so creating the experience of control. This does not mean closing an interview abruptly, as moving into the closing stages needs to be a gradual process. It may be useful to highlight this by warning the patient that it is time to begin drawing the interview to a close and therefore necessary to collect thoughts and feelings together. It is rarely necessary to extend the time limit, although the counsellor may feel a little heartless drawing a consultation to an end when a patient is very distressed. However, complex or disturbing interviews can be continued at another time. The counsellor may find something like the following phrase useful: 'We've covered a lot of upsetting issues today and we need to allow time for you to think about the issues raised, so we'll continue when we next meet'.

Ending a consultation is the ability to say goodbye and to leave the patient to their family and friends for support or even to manage alone. The same process of ending and saying goodbye happens when a series of interviews has ended, or when a long supportive relationship is closed. In both these circumstances the counsellor has to be able to let go and allow the patient to find their own way. Ending a difficult and upsetting interview gives the patient the message that they are capable of managing their upset. This is sometimes difficult for a counsellor who wants to ease a person's pain and make things better. The ease or difficulty with which a consultation can be ended is a reflection of individual difference in attachment patterns. The individual with a secure attachment is able to manage separation and will be able to leave to continue any emotional tasks alone or with outside support. However when an individual has an insecure attachment pattern, the emotions, dilemma and counsellor will be dealt with either dismissively or very anxiously. In the same way the nature of the counsellor's attachment pattern will also affect how an interview is ended. The secure counsellor will be able to let a patient go with compassion and sadness and allow the patient to carry their own pain; the insecure dismissive will avoid the significance and end the interview without compassion whilst the insecure preoccupied will cling to the patient, allowing them to go beyond the allotted time and trying to be more and more helpful.

The psychological space

The psychological space exists in the relationship developed between the patient and the counsellor (which in attachment terms is the secure-enough base). The quality of that professional relationship determines the creative potential for sharing feelings, developing thinking and decision-making. The counsellor has to combine education and facilitation and is challenged to structure an interview appropriately. There are facts to understand and a history to be established alongside giving time and space for exploring feelings and developing thinking. However, even when giving information the counsellor is taking account of the patient's responses and adjusting accordingly. This ensures that the psychological space is always kept alive.

In some disorders, such as cancer and Huntington's disease, protocols have been introduced where the implications of being tested are considered over a series of consultations. These can be very constructive as they ensure that all aspects are covered. However, there is a danger that the actual content of the interview is structured to such a degree that inexperienced counsellors will not allow enough space for spontaneous thoughts and ideas to emerge. The psychological space is then squeezed out. Further, the inexperienced counsellor may confuse the educative and facilitating approaches. In the former, issues are raised by an active counsellor; in the latter, psychological issues are allowed to emerge and the counsellor's activity is one of listening and waiting. The knowledge that certain feelings can arise may lead an inexperienced counsellor to ask questions such as, 'Are you feeling guilty or depressed?' Alternatively the counsellor may treat the psychological issues in an educative manner by informing that depression or guilt may occur. These approaches are well-meaning and attempt to make sure that nothing is missed but they interfere with the internal processes of the patient. With experience the counsellor learns to listen for the emotions and only name what is there. To raise them is like giving a patient a list of side effects which are then looked for. The psychological space is kept open by the counsellor being aware and considering how the patient is registering the experience.

The elements of a therapeutic professional relationship
The 'facilitating environment' and 'potential space'

Winnicott (1971) and Bion (1959) developed an in-depth understanding of the conditions necessary to develop a therapeutic encounter. Both developed their ideas from an understanding of the mother/infant relationship and applied it to the therapeutic encounter. Winnicott used the terms 'facilitating environment and good-enough mother'; Bion used 'the container and the contained' to refer to a particular quality and nature of the mother/infant relationship. In the last chapter the importance of the relationship between the mother and infant was discussed in the development of the secure base in the professional encounter. All these terms are used to describe the same qualities and as they are all used it is important for the counsellor to be familiar with their meaning. Winnicott's explorations of the mother and infant identified the 'good-enough' mother as having particular qualities – an attitude of being emotionally available, supportive, aware and understanding of the infant's vulnerability. Winnicott (1988) used the term 'holding' to refer to the actual physical holding of the infant by the mother and also the emotional holding of attunement in the mother's mind. That relationship could then become 'facilitating' for emotional growth and development. These ideas can be transferred to a professional consultation and the empathic understanding of a patient's anxiety. Winnicott emphasised that constructive relaxation could take place in the confidence of a living relationship. Further a well-timed interpretation of correct understanding 'gives a sense of being held, that is more real than if a real holding had taken place'. However, he points out how this can be interfered with if there is anxiety in the caregiver.

The term 'potential space' is related to the 'facilitating environment' and is the interactional space created within the relationship. It is a shared space where the conversation takes place and an understanding of each other can be achieved. It refers to the potential for exploration, thought and creativity to develop when there is a degree of confidence, trust, interest and reliability in the relationship. Winnicott quotes the importance of the capacity of 'if I were in your shoes …' and in so doing is pointing out that the essential ingredient in establishing a 'facilitating environment' with 'potential space' is empathy.

In a similar way, Bion (1959) also explored the mother/infant relationship and applied it to the professional relationship. There are however some additional ideas which relate to what happens as a result of the mother being attuned to the infant's vulnerable, anxious self. Bion used the terms 'contained' by the 'container' to describe the process of anxiety being understood (contained), by the container (the mother). More importantly, the mother is capable of transforming the anxious or angry negative emotions of the infant and giving them back in a positive form. In everyday life this happens when a mother is heard lovingly saying to her screaming infant, 'Oh, dear you are so upset, you are tired …' In the professional relationship the terms refer to the ability of the counsellor to tolerate negative emotions, to be able to internally process them and transform them into positive feelings of empathy, concern and compassion. In practice, the counsellor is not disturbed by the patient's high anxiety, but understands the fear, is able to tolerate it and gently and compassionately conveys that sentiment. In a more contractual language the counsellor and patient have to set up a working alliance.

The working alliance

This term refers to the necessity for the counsellor and patient to work together to complete the agreed tasks. The ease or difficulty of forming an alliance is related to the attachment pattern of the patient. The counsellor recognises the different attachment patterns by listening to the patient's language, tracking the content and meaning, and assessing the patient's style of handling their story and emotions. These factors help the counsellor determine what adjustments need to be made to create an effective professional relationship. The counsellor's sensitivity to the individual's style is a determining factor in development of a working alliance. Bordin (1982) considers that there are three components to the working alliance: a consensus between the counsellor and patient on the goals of the encounter; an agreement on the topics and number of meetings to address how the goal is achieved; and, most importantly, the development of a strong affective bond between the professional and patient.

The co-construction of purpose of an interview with the definition of roles

A natural corollary to the working alliance is the idea of the co-construction of the purpose of the interview where the counsellor and patient jointly agree on the purpose of the interview. This usually happens at the beginning of an interview with the counsellor exploring who is asking what question. The following two examples demonstrate different styles of clarifying the purpose of the consultation.

Examples

1. In this example the counsellor actually states the focus early in the consultation. There has been a clarification of the patient's request and the counsellor continues by saying, 'We're going to think about quite a lot in the next hour and we're going to try and give you the information you need …. There are a lot of steps to go through in the next hour and what I want to find out is, if after having all the information, you want to know whether if the predisposition for cancer in the family has come down to you', or 'We are going to discuss the possibility of having blood tests for the bowel cancer that is in the family'. These statements give the focus, aim and time frame, thus telling the patient exactly what is going to happen.

2. In contrast, the following example is taken from an extract of a pure counselling consultation. The focus and role is set within the conversation and demonstrates that even in a session where the task is less crisply defined, there is still an identification of roles and focusing of the interview.

Extract

A man requested an interview as he felt he was not coping with his diagnosis and the problems it had generated. He began by saying he was not certain why he had come and the counsellor replied that there had been an idea that he might want to talk. The patient continued by agreeing and saying that he needed to talk to a stranger so that he could 'rabbit on' as he was worried about hurting family or boring friends. He continued by saying, 'I wanted to talk to someone I didn't know. It's difficult to express your feelings with people you know. So you tend to bottle things up. That's why I asked for this counselling … I don't know whether what I'm going through is the same as what other people go through. You don't want to keep talking about feelings so people think you feel sorry for yourself'.

The patient had identified the task by explaining he wanted to talk differently, differentiating ordinary conversation from professional conversation. He also clarified his need to express feelings and thus defined the function of the interview. He was looking for similarities and differences, searching for patterns, wondering whether he was on a normal path. Implied in this statement is the idea that the counsellor would be able to help in these ways and so positions 'a giver' and 'a receiver'.

The counsellor responded by using a metaphor, 'You are not sure how much of the stage to take in ordinary conversation, feeling you might be taking centre stage inappropriately with friends, whereas here it is different'. The patient eagerly agreed and laughingly said, 'I suppose you have to listen to me, that's your job'.

Here the counsellor responded to the patient's need to talk by using the metaphor of the stage which suggests that there was a script, where one was the speaker and the other the listener. In this short space of time the counsellor and patient had defined their focus, purpose and also their roles, allowing the interview to continue.

Although it is important for the counsellor to allow considerable space for the patient to tell their story, it is the counsellor's job to keep the focus, not rigidly but to hold the discussion to the task in hand. Sometimes, it may be difficult to interrupt a patient who is telling a personally significant and painful story (and indeed it may well be relevant to the genetic story), but with skill and experience the counsellor will be able to balance listening to the story and focusing on the genetic task. Individuals with an insecure, preoccupied attachment pattern sometimes get lost in the story or their emotional upset and may need the counsellor to interrupt. Comments such as 'I know we have come to a painful point in the story, but let's try and return to the questions you were asking at the beginning of the session', so gently, yet authoritatively, returning to the task.

Empathy

Empathy is a 'feeling state' of being able to understand someone else's subjective experience and is the essential skill in human interaction. In writing about empathy Pines (1993) quotes Condon (1984), a leading figure in communication research, as stating that 'empathy and communication are fundamental to human life and that we are highly complex centres of communication, common beings with many forms of sharing with fellow human beings in a common world'. Pines provides the literal meaning of empathy as 'in-feeling, feeling into', but clarifies that it is only one aspect of the empathic process as there are two facets, an active and a passive version. The active is the entering into the other; the passive is giving oneself up to the other, allowing the experience of the other to enter. The active form involves the desire to understand and explore the experience of the other with imagination; the passive necessitates a self-negation and an openness to receive the experience of the other.

Empathy is the *sine qua non* of a therapeutic encounter as it enables two people to experience the pain of one. It is the ingredient the counsellor needs to establish the secure base referred to in attachment theory; the factor required to establish the 'facilitating environment' with 'potential space' (Winnicott, 1971); and the necessary ingredient for containment (Bion, 1962).

Empathy needs to be differentiated from sympathy which is the compassionate feeling for, or with another, involving closeness and warmth which is highly personalised. Empathy is objective and more separate, and although it involves personal or professional intimacy, it acknowledges that the experience belongs to the other and not to the self. There is therefore a feeling *into*, rather than *with* an individual. It is understanding the subjective experience of the other, which is different from the recalling a similar personal experience. To achieve this special form of communication, the counsellor has to suspend personal ideas and views to be receptive, linked and attuned to the patient in order to understand the other person's mindset.

Although empathy is a feeling state it becomes a very subtle tool which the counsellor uses to reach the patient whilst maintaining an observer self. The counsellor is affected, but is not identified with, or overwhelmed by the other's reality. This challenges counsellors to be aware of their own emotions and to be wary of counselling a patient who has similar personal difficulties. For instance, it would be difficult if the counsellor had suffered a recent bereavement to be therapeutically available to a patient who was also grieving. The personal preoccupation could prevent the counsellor being comfortable enough to be able to sit with someone else's anxiety without over-identifying, becoming defensive, or confused about who owns what emotion. The counsellor needs to be secure enough to be both in the interaction and outside, which is above or 'meta' to the interaction. This involves experiencing the patient's reality, observing the personal experience and the interaction, as if having one foot in the exchange and another outside. It is as if there is a third person in the room. This situation actually happens when the counsellor relays the details of the counselling session to a supervisor. The counselling session is brought alive in the presence of a third person, the supervisor. With ongoing supervision the counsellor internalises the ideas created in a supervision experience. This can develop into having the supervisor in mind whilst counselling so that an internal supervisor or third person is then present in all consultations.

Empathy not only has active and passive elements, but also sensory and motor components of understanding and conveying that understanding. The sensory component involves understanding the other's subjective experience but, this is not enough, as the counsellor has to personally process the experience to fully understand and then use the motor component to convey that understanding. This means that the counsellor moves into and out of the patient's experience, personally processing the emotions and then giving the experience back to the patient in a different way. The manner of conveying an empathic understanding involves tact. This has the quality of knowing how far to go and, if it is gauged correctly, can create the experience of a soothing touch; whereas if misjudged it can be intrusive and exposing. Pines (1993) considers that the professional's awareness of personal shame is a key factor in guiding the counsellor towards this balance.

In the following example a clinician inadvertently uses a diagnosis and, as a result, it has a serious effect on the mother and how she perceived her child.

Example

Two sisters from a family, where four generations have Saethre–Chotzen syndrome, have varying degrees of facial changes. The more severely affected woman has a child with minimal facial changes and she believes her child is free of the condition; the less affected sister has a child with very marked facial changes and the diagnosis is acknowledged. The first woman had been teased at school and was pleased that she had what she had thought was a normal child who would not have her painful experience in school. She consulted a clinician when her child had an unrelated problem and, in that consultation, the clinician remarked, 'I see he has Chotzen syndrome like his cousin'. In a stroke the child was transformed in the mother's eyes and had become 'diseased like me'.

A more aware clinician would have had some thoughts of, 'I wonder what it must be like for this woman to be confronted with her disorder reflected in her child's face'. That thought alone would have inhibited the statement and the empathic attunement would have protected the mother, but its absence shocked her and exposed what she did not want to see.

This is the type of unwitting remark we are all guilty of at some point in time. It illustrates how the function and meaning of a diagnosis is regarded differently by clinicians and patients. For the clinician it is an example of clinical diagnostic expertise and enables any treatment plan to be put in place; in the mother's eyes it confers a different identity on the child and predicts a different future. The mother had been using the defence of denial which had constructively allowed her to see her child as normal and different from her. Suddenly, that defence had been shattered and she became seriously disturbed. The woman, who had found a way of dealing with her difficulties which had protected her child, was unprepared for the uninvited diagnostic labelling. As a result, she had to adjust to the diagnosis she was avoiding. Clearly the experience was traumatic and, in addition, it has the potential to alter her perception of her child and the relationship between them.

The understanding of empathy and containment can be expanded by referring to Dennett (1983) who clarifies that containment refers to the mother's capacity to contain the infant by responding emotionally in a manner that modulates unmanageable feelings, and acknowledges the child's 'intentional stance'. This means that the mother reflects both the cause of the distress and her appreciation of the affective state of the child (Fonagy, 1995). This emphasises that empathy and containment go beyond mirroring (Meltzoff and Gopnik, 1993), as the caregiver reflects the child's emotional state and her own adult mastery of it. Fonagy (1995) points out that going beyond mirroring implies that the caregiver has the capacity not to be overwhelmed by the distress, but can deal with it. In applying this to the therapeutic encounter it alerts the counsellor to an awareness of their own ability to withstand anxiety and to tolerate negativity before they can be an effective container for a patient.

From the idea of containment, Bion's work gives an understanding of thinking processes and how unprocessed emotions interfere with the ability to take in information and think. This theoretical point is of considerable interest for genetic counselling.

Facilitating thinking

It has been emphasised how anxiety interferes with decision-making and how the task of the patient is to contain extremes of emotion to aid decision-making and to process the effects of a result. The counsellor becomes involved in helping with this process, especially when the patient has an insecure attachment pattern and is unable to successfully manage the emotions. The containment of anxiety is a core element of a genetic consultation. It relates to the ability to think in a way which involves the linkage of ideas and the ability to deduce meaning such that one way of measuring the success of the counselling encounter would be to reach a point when the individual can think clearly. In Bion's model, the precursor of this capacity is related to the mother's capacity to contain and process the infant's chaotic experiences and to make sense of them. The mother understands the infant's distress by conveying an understanding of the emotion and the intent or desire. In conveying this, her words and tone change the infant's experience and converts distress into rest or pleasure. From this observation, Bion differentiated these two states of mind-chaos and calm. He explained that the movement from the one to the other took place by the distress of anxiety being contained by understanding and, as a result, the distress is given shape, form and meaning. It is transformed. As a result bad experiences do not need to be got rid of, but can be digested and thought about. The main result in this process is the ability to tolerate frustration and grief such that pain or anxiety can be faced and fully felt.

Transferring this idea to genetic counselling, the counsellor knows that by containing the patient's anxiety, understanding the experience and the intent, the patient will be helped to think, achieve a reflective state of mind and consider the dilemma creatively. Most people will have some personal experience of the difference between these two states of mind. For example, at one moment it is possible to feel very panicky, unable to face an issue, or in everyday language 'feel all over the place'; at another moment the anxiety settles and can be replaced by a feeling of quiet sadness. When sadness is fully felt, the individual can feel the pain, know what it is, yet feel perfectly integrated and able to consider and think. This change demonstrates the movement from chaos to calm through the containment of extreme emotions to feel constructively sad. In contrast when anxiety, confusion, unprocessed grief or other experiences are undigested, an agitated state of mind is created. Under those circumstances, thoughts are fragmented and not linked and information cannot be taken in. The individual, either literally or metaphorically, resorts to running around in circles, blocking or splitting off thoughts.

Bion expanded further by describing how under certain conditions, it is possible to take in information, assess a situation accurately, think clearly and make decisions. He related that to the processing of emotions. In that frame of mind, the individual is able to self-reflect, which means not only experiencing, but also thinking about the experience. The ability to self-reflect results in both experiencing an 'I' and thinking about a 'me'. With that ability, it is possible for anxiety to be controlled as the individual can think 'I feel anxious', and 'this is me feeling anxious'. In that state, thoughts are linked and there is consistency, where an internal wisdom is created and emotions and cognitions are integrated. The genetic counsellor can detect this in someone by recognising that the individual is demonstrating a more balanced outlook and is able to consider the whole picture. At that moment the individual is emotionally aware, yet able to be objective about the self. The following example is an extract from an interview of a patient who is self-reflecting and considering differences over time.

Extract

When I was first told I was all over the place, I was frightened. I'd wake up in the morning and think 'has it gone away?' Then I'd realise, 'no it hasn't.' I'd try and hide from it by staying in bed and if I got up, I couldn't eat, I felt so sick. Now I'm different, I'm sort of older, sort of more sober. I can't say I'm happy but I manage and I can talk about it now'. The patient continued, 'I'm different now you know, or I think I am, and so, in a sense, it's like an ego boost for me to tell you what I've done and I haven't done…. In a sense it's not an ego boost as such, but at least by talking about it, it sort of brings it back on myself… and what I've been through and coped with is always wondering and considering what an individual is asking or trying to say'.

The patient insightfully comments that in talking about his difficulty and thinking about differences over time he says 'it brings it back on him'. He is thinking aloud, reflecting, integrating and also assessing his present position and comparing it to his former self. His self-reflection gives him an overview and a deeper understanding.

Communicative competence and listening skills of integrating meaning

The theoretical points discussed in this chapter have looked the structure of the interview and the nature of the counselling relationship. There are additional factors which need to be considered and these are related to the idea of communicative competence. The communicative competence of the counsellor is the ability to listen and hear not just content, but also to what has so far been called 'intent'. Another way of understanding what is meant by 'intent' is to consider the meaning of what is being said. This is important for the genetic counsellor who understands the patient's distress by conveying an understanding of the emotion, and the intent or desire. In a discourse study of 'good' and 'poor' communication in medical students, Roberts et al. (2003) structured clinical examination and teased out different communicative styles between the two groups. They found these were related to the use of empathy, the ability to build up a theme in stages (as opposed to introducing a theme too early) and the beliefs values and ideologies held about their relationships with patients. The students presented themselves on a spectrum that stretched from a position of personal authority and conviction to a reliance on medical evidence and procedures. The authors considered that a balance between the two seemed the most successful. Applying this to genetic counselling would translate as the counsellor integrating the educational and emotional styles.

A considerable amount of genetic counselling is rightly about giving information in the form of explanations and this fulfils the need for the patient to understand. Sarangi (2000), after studying transcripts of genetic counselling sessions, pointed out that the counsellor used explanations in response to requests for information or advice. He likened the interaction to a lecturer–student interaction which he stated is different from mainstream doctor–patient interaction. At another point, he commented that if information is a commodity, the exchange corresponded to a service encounter. In his analysis the discourse type was not a straight information-giving exercise, but was packaged into 'modes of explanation' using statements, classification, causes and the deployment of metaphors.

The basic elements of communication in a professional encounter include turn-taking, listening and speaking. The counsellor identifies key words used by the patient and follows or tracks the train of thought, joins with the style of thinking by speaking in a way which incorporates similar words or thinking processes. The counsellor is also reading the non-verbal behaviour and considering the level of intelligence.

The risk in genetic counselling is that the counsellor relies too heavily on educative interventions and gives too much information, or uses explanations to address emotional issues and does not pay enough attention to the relationship with the patient. A number of words such as 'joining', 'mutuality', 'attunement' and 'empathy' have been used to describe the effective professional relationship. To illustrate further it can be likened to a dance where the task of the professional is to be 'in step' with the patient and not vice versa. The inexperienced genetic counsellor can fall 'out of step' with the patient by not being emotionally attuned, or alternatively the counsellor can dictate the dance by allowing the educative stance to dominate. Equally, a patient cannot be allowed to dominate. There needs to be a mutual awareness, one with another, of being 'in step' and then something creative can happen and the patient is more likely to absorb information as a result.

As a consultation proceeds, a counsellor may be alerted to the meaning of the request being different from the surface content and this takes the understanding of communication to another level. Indeed, it can be useful to regard a request for a genetic consultation as an entry point and, unconsciously, the genetic problem may be a convenient ticket of entry for a discussion. The experienced counsellor will have seen many requests for genetic counselling which are covers for a variety of problems and these can become revealed in the consultation.

Sometimes the counsellor does not hear the meaning of what the patient is trying to say and the progress of an interview may then be blocked. One sign that this is happening is an interactional sequence being repeated many times and this is demonstrated in the next example. It shows how useful explanations can be, but also how a patient who repeatedly asks questions is also making a statement. If the counsellor stays in an educative mode, then the meaning of the repeated questioning is not heard. However the interview changes when the counsellor engages more empathically and demonstrates that the patient's underlying emotional distress has been heard.

Example

A patient, who was intellectually very well-informed, asked for more and more information about a heart condition which had affected her father. She asked numerous questions in quick succession, all of which were looking for advice on how she and her young daughter should live their lives, given that she might have inherited the disorder. Each time she was given the correct factual answer and on a number of occasions she commented in a questioning way 'I can't take any reassurance from that'. The counsellor continued to respond to each question by giving the explanatory answers in a very thoughtful manner but did not attend to the comment. The question, answer and comment became a repeated pattern, as if the patient was going through a checklist and looking for a reassuring answer.

The consultation was interrupted and, after the break, the counsellor then wisely took the opportunity to summarise the consultation. Included in the summary were the facts of the history, the information about the disorder and the fact that the woman was anxious for herself and for her child. The counsellor speculated that the woman's intention was to cover all aspects of the disorder and to know as much as possible. By acknowledging the disorder, having the appropriate investigations, accessing monitoring and following correct advice about diet and exercise, she would be doing her best to deal with the worry. As the counsellor conveyed an understanding of the woman's emotional state and her intentions, the pattern and mood of the interview changed. The patient responded by being more relaxed and open and dropped her repeated questioning. The counsellor had included in the summary an awareness of the patient's urgency and search for reassurance and consequently integrated the educative and emotional aspects around the disorder. As a result, the woman felt understood; she could give up her repeated questioning.

In this example the counsellor revealed a more complete understanding by pausing and summarising, as if discussing the consultation in a supervision session. The counsellor had developed an ability to be in the interaction and outside it, describing it as if a third person were in the room. This is the self-reflective position described earlier, with the counsellor having an awareness of 'I am doing this' and 'This is me doing this'; the most constructive position for the counsellor.

Alternatively, in this example, the counsellor could have used the technique of empathising and including the intent or meaning of the patient's thinking. The patient gave a number of clues that she is looking for reassurance both in her search for more information, but also in her comments. An empathic approach would have included something like – 'I can hear that you are looking for some reassurance and that you are trying to do the right things to avoid the trouble your father had'.

Another approach would involve the counsellor looking at the interactional dynamic which was repeated. As the counsellor tried harder and harder, with infinite patience, to answer all the questions, it led to more of the same so creating an underlying tension and frustration in the dynamic. In contrast, acknowledging the dynamic could result in something like, 'It seems that I can't quite leave you feeling you have all the information you would like. Let's see if you can tell me what I am missing out?' To address all of these points (integrating the information seeking, the underlying anxiety and the pattern of interaction between patient and counsellor) would mean saying something like: 'You are desperately trying to understand this condition and as a result of receiving the information you are learning a lot. But, I suspect that when I try to give you the relevant information, even though it is useful, I am also missing something out as we are not talking about how anxious you are and how worried you are that your son might have this disorder'. This statement includes a summary of the content, an overview of the interaction and contains an acknowledgement of the underlying anxiety (with the search for reassurance), as well as the desires of both professional and patient.

Communication is at varying levels; a basic level of listening, tracking and turn-taking. This reaches another level when refined by the more personal communication of empathic understanding – thus adding the dimension of a thoughtful and kind human encounter. If the counsellor can understand the underlying intention then the interaction is more than mirroring. It is true empathy. This last element adds the dimension of understanding the hidden meaning of the interaction. Adding all these elements makes an enormous difference which can be likened to the difference between an ordinary musician who has mastered the technique and someone who conveys a deep understanding of the music.

It is interesting that, in a supervision session, the counsellor often reveals more psychological awareness and intuition than is used in the clinical encounter. It is difficult to know whether this is a question of the counsellor's confidence in addressing psychological issues, or whether the counsellor is so intent on doing a good job of giving explanations and information, that the awareness or sensitivity to the meaning is kept at the back of the mind and not always integrated. It may therefore be useful to adopt the technique of summarising or giving a formulation to include the psychological insights. This self-reflective way of conversing triggers self-reflection in the patient, it models the possibility of the patient both feeling and thinking about feeling which is the ideal state of mind for a genetic consultation.

The use of metaphor

We use metaphors in our everyday speech; there are metaphors that we live by and invariably the meaning is understood. It is use of a particular kind of language which brings with it pictures, colours, stories and seems to be immediately understood by everyone. Metaphorical language is a poetic language, very different from logical or scientific speech, one which we seem programmed to understand. It is a language which is often used in psychotherapy.

Metaphor language can be important in the genetic counsellor's clinical practice. It can facilitate an understanding where logical thought, clarification or explanation has failed. It allows difficult ideas, concepts or problems to be spoken about in a tangential manner, when a more direct approach would be too anxiety provoking. To be accurate and effective, it must refer precisely to the individual, but the essence of a metaphor is that it applies universally and therefore not specifically to the individual.

Metaphorical language involves a leap in thinking into the realm of imagination to play with ideas. It appears to be a shared language, mutually understood and is therefore a very easy way of joining with a patient's experience. Something is captured which is universally recognisable through an image which acts as a vehicle carrying meaning. The literal paraphrasing of a metaphor is often a long explanation which fails to excite or ignite the imagination of the individual. The effect of literal language is different from the effect of metaphorical language. Literal language is logical; metaphorical language needs no logic, its meaning is conveyed in the story or image.

Metaphors can be used in any number of ways and fulfil a number of functions: to join with the patient and convey understanding, to reframe, to explain, explore, confront, etc. Metaphors can be introduced by a patient or a counsellor and are successful when understood by both.

In genetic counselling most of the time the language is literal, giving information, but when talking about certain genetic inheritance patterns, the counsellor frequently explains it as having either a 'single' or 'double dose' of a gene, or the counsellor might liken genetic inheritance to the 'toss of a coin'. Metaphorical language can therefore be a bridge linking the literal information with everyday speech to illustrate a point.

The following examples show how metaphors can be used in a number of different ways.

1. In an initial consultation a patient was exploring being tested for the gene linked to the bowel cancer in his family. At a thoughtful moment the patient said, 'You see, this isn't easy to decide, as I normally sit on the fence'. The counsellor was able to use this metaphor and invited him to imagine what it would be like to be on different sides

of the fence. Later it was acknowledged that although sitting on the fence protected him from making a decision, it was also a painful position to be in. Here, the counsellor stays with what is essentially a dead metaphor and gives it life by asking the patient to imagine being on first one then the other side of the fence. The counsellor then makes a change by moving to the literal experience by saying how sitting on the fence can also be painful. This refers to the literal and physical experience, but the meaning that avoidance is painful is included. The desirability of making a decision is therefore spoken about, without it being directly addressed.

2. A woman, in her twenties, was struggling with the conflict of whether to be tested for the Huntington's disease gene which was in her family. She explained she would not have children if she tested positive for the gene, and that there was conflict between her and her husband around her being tested before becoming pregnant. Her husband would not speak about it, except to say to his wife that he would not be able to cope if he could not have children. She was finding the conflict so disturbing that it was interfering with her every thought. Her conclusion was to be tested immediately and not to tell her husband. She found the counselling very difficult and just wanted to be tested and not discuss anything. The counsellor explained why there was a protocol of several consultations and tried to help her consider speaking to her husband further. She was invited to consider the effects of counselling on herself, her husband and their relationship but was unable to respond to any of the counsellor's interventions. The situation changed when the counsellor used a metaphor saying, 'You seem to be in a "Catch 22" position'. The woman became upset and spoke more openly about the conflict. On the one hand, she risked alienating her husband; on the other hand, she felt she would be irresponsible to become pregnant without testing.

The interview progressed but she still wanted to be tested immediately. She could not imagine talking further and had no hope of resolving the conflict. The counsellor then used another metaphor, saying, 'It seems as if the only way you can deal with this difficulty is to grit your teeth and jump as if off a high diving board. The woman laughed and said, 'I might do myself an injury if I'm not careful'. They both laughingly played with this idea and developed the suggestions that she ought to make sure that there was water in the pool, and that she could swim. The first metaphor had enabled the counsellor to join with her dilemma; the second to overcome a difficulty. She subsequently agreed to an appointment for both her and her husband with the counsellor.

In this example a patient, who is very frightened and stuck, is helped to think about the problem she cannot consider in logical thought as it makes her too anxious. The use of the metaphor allowed her to acknowledge that she was not prepared. It also side-stepped the process of becoming more intense and serious, or giving more information, trying to use reason.

3. In the following example a metaphor is used to encourage a patient who was finding it difficult to adjust to the knowledge of having the gene for bowel cancer.

   In an upset manner a man said, 'I'm so angry and depressed I can't get myself going to get the tests done. I find it such hard work and I don't feel I'm not making any progress.' The counsellor replied, 'You are working very hard and maybe you are well on the road. You may need to think about the tortoise and the hare, as the tortoise did rather well in my storybook'. This brought considerable laughter and a response from the patient of 'I'll press on then'. A more straightforward approach would have been for the counsellor to be reassuring and comment, 'You are doing well'. The metaphor did that work and encouraged in a way that predicted winning the battle. More importantly the patient found his own direction.

4. This next example reveals how a metaphor can be used to express a difficulty central to genetic counselling. A middle-aged single woman, unable to decide whether to go ahead with testing for the Huntington's gene, says 'I don't know what to do, I don't know which way to turn, it's as if I'm at a crossroad'. She continued, 'I don't know where I'm meant to go, which is the right way to go?' The counsellor replied 'You speak as if there were a map and a right road and I guess you'd like someone to show you which way to go. The problem is you can go down either road and that's the difficulty. Let's imagine you are making a journey down each one in turn and let's see what it might be like to travel down either road. I'll try and accompany you, let's see where we get to'.

5. A young woman had been investigated for her repeated miscarriages and was again pregnant. She began the consultation with a metaphor, 'I'm not in a very nice place' and explained how she was unable to do anything, did not want to go out, rejected friends and did not know what she wanted. She felt she ought to be happy as she was pregnant but she was not.

   The counsellor invited her to picture her difficulty. She responded by saying she felt paralysed and just did not know. The counsellor commented that she seemed stuck, in a sort of limbo. The woman was able to say more about how she felt and replied that she was certainly waiting, but she did not know whether it was for, something good or bad, 'Heaven or Hell'. She continued 'That's it exactly. Am I waiting for a baby? Or to be told it's not possible'.

   The mood of this interview was changed by the use of the idea of limbo. The patient had previously been unable to say very much, other than speak about her low mood. The idea of limbo captured her imagination and enabled her to crystallise her dilemma. She understood she was neither in Heaven nor Hell, a thought which released her to verbalise her position more clearly.

6. The following extract is part of the end of a consultation where a patient had been discussing the major changes needed to adapt to a new way of living. In the extract,

the patient and counsellor are reflecting together. The patient is a teacher and the counsellor designs a relevant metaphor to understand the idea of adjustment as building up words and progressing educationally.

C: You have been telling me about all the changes you have had to make to adjust to the way you have to live now you have this problem. You are going into the world where you are at the beginning of learning something new.
P: Effectively, I think so.

C: How fluent and confident do you feel in what we might say is a new language? Are you at the stage of learning the alphabet the a b c of the basics of how life might be, or are you further and can put words together to make sentences?
P: I can put sentences together but they are quiet simple. I guess the fluency will come with practice. And then I'll know the meaning as well.

Later in the same consultation the patient reflects, 'I've learned a lot, finding my way in the world again, but it's a bit like being a child again'. The counsellor picks up the patient's idea and elaborates, 'well it is and it isn't in that now you may be learning lots of new things, but now you are learning with the skills of an adult. You are may feel like a child, overwhelmed, but with the skills of an adult you can learn quickly'.

In this extract the counsellor is inviting the patient to reflect on the progress and the use of the metaphor allows it to be understood as a developmental process which, although new, can be approached with the experience of an adult.

Reflecting on these examples the use of metaphor takes the patient and counsellor away from the direct problem to look at it in another way, which is not personal, yet encapsulates their dilemma. The individual is somehow freed and can begin to think about themselves, instead of being stuck or overwhelmed by their problem.

From a psychotherapeutic view point the use of metaphor creates a potential space for playing with ideas. It uses another medium, a poetic or narrative language.

This chapter has demonstrated the importance of the counsellor understanding the patient and using it in both the educative and more facilitating aspects of the counselling process. The counsellor has to straddle the fence of following the patient's lead whilst also guiding the interview appropriately. The skills from psychotherapy help the counsellor act like a conductor of an orchestra, setting boundaries, entering the patient's experience and holding the whole experience together.

Summary points

The empathic skills of the counsellor involve creating a physical and psychological space which is a facilitating environment for the patient. When the counsellor understands the patient's subjective experience and the intentional stance, anxiety is contained.

The containment of anxiety transforms the chaotic experience of very high anxiety and enables the patient to think, make decisions, process emotions and tolerate frustration.

The accurate use of metaphorical language can convey empathy, clarify confusion, confront difficulties and resolve conflict. Correctly designed it applies to the individual yet is understood as having a universal meaning.

Examples of the role and skills of the counsellor

In the first half of this book a framework has been presented which enables the genetic counsellor to think about genetic counselling in terms of stress theory, coping and the use of defences. It has also used attachment theory and ideas from psychotherapy to guide the counsellor's understanding of the patient, the interview process and the appropriate therapeutic response. This chapter presents clinical examples to focus in more detail on extracts from clinical practice to give the reader a better feel for integrating these theoretical points.

Working with anxiety and grief

The next three examples demonstrate the importance of containing anxiety and processing grief to facilitate a different way of thinking as explained in the discussion of empathy and, in particular, Bion's work on facilitating thinking.

Working with anxiety and a changing state of mind

It is very common in genetic counselling for a patient to enter the consulting room in a highly charged emotional state and, as explained, that interferes with the ability to take in the whole picture and consider the issues comprehensively. Frequently, there will be a sense of urgency and agitation about a person whose mind cannot be still enough to process the complexities arising. As the woman in this example explains, successful genetic counselling creates a space for the patient to listen and take in information, express any relevant upset and be able to settle down to consider the issue in hand.

Example

In a cancer genetic interview a patient says: 'I understand a bit better now. . . . When I was first in the room, I thought, oh let's get this over quick like, I was spinning and wanted to run. It all seemed so awful, my mother and my sister dying and me thinking it was me next. But you've slowed me down a bit, I've cried too. I never thought I would, but I understand a bit more and it might not be my turn next. But if it is, then I'd better find out and then think about what I need to do next, I suppose it's not all hopeless'.

From this transcript it would seem that the counsellor has given information to the patient which clarified a number of emotive issues about the relevant risk. In addition, in the interview, there has been space and time for the woman to express and work through her upset. Her words: 'you've slowed me down' suggest an important relationship was established between her and the counsellor. As a result, the woman was able to have a different perspective on her dilemma. She had benefited from the counsellor integrating the educative and emotional aspects of the problem. When this happens it brings a sense of freedom and lightness to the interview.

Entering the fear

Individuals are sometimes frightened of being frightened and think that they will not be able to cope. This state of high anxiety can result in a feeling of chaos and panic in which the thinking processes are interrupted as explained by Bion (1959). Under that circumstance the patient often avoids the feared area. However, if the counsellor can enter the feared area by being interested to understand, the patient can be helped to contain the anxiety. Acknowledging the anxiety and confronting the fears makes them more manageable. This process is demonstrated in the following extract.

Extract

A man, who was considering being tested for Huntington's disease, insightfully said, 'I put on a brave face and I tell everyone I would manage if I had a bad result, but that's a lie, I don't know what I would do'.

The counsellor picked up this statement of 'not knowing what he would do' as it suggested extreme panic and a fear that he felt he could not cope. The counsellor replied, 'You say you don't know what you would do but, I wonder if what you are saying is that you would be extremely frightened and confused. Tell me how you imagine you would be or, what comes to mind when you think about the possibility'. The man replied, 'I remember what my mother was like, it was awful and I just want to curl up and disappear when I think of her. This illness is disgusting; no one should have to suffer such a degrading death. No dignity, I don't want that. There's nothing I can do about it and I don't know how much I will know about how bad I am. I don't usually talk about this, it's too awful and now I've said it'. At that point he laughed. The counsellor replied 'It sounds as if that memory of your mother was haunting you and, I wonder if those sorts of fears need to see the light of day, rather than be locked up inside you'. The man continued, 'Well I hope I haven't got it, but if I have, I won't have any children, I couldn't do that to them. I don't want to burden my wife, so that's another reason for knowing, so I can find a way of getting care, so her life isn't ruined as well'.

The counsellor replied, 'You said earlier you don't know what you would do, and yet, you've clearly thought about all the possible scenarios. So although it's all very frightening and, as you say, you feel powerless, you have actually made a lot of plans which is, in fact, coping. But, I guess you are also saying you are very frightened and don't know how to solve the problem such that it goes away'. 'That's it exactly', he replied.

In this interview the man revealed what was behind his public face of coping and revealed his fear of not coping. The counsellor skilfully helped him enter his area of dread and what emerged was the figure of his mother and her suffering (and his nightmare of being like his mother). Although this may not take away the fear, talking about it, by giving words to what seems unthinkable, gives chaos and terror a form. Terror had become manageable fear. The unthinkable had been looked at, expressed and then, thought about.

Working with unresolved grief to facilitate thinking

This is another example of an interactional sequence being repeated where a patient, in a very agitated state of mind, was unable to hear the meaning of the counsellor's educative intervention (this suggests that there is some emotion which is unprocessed and blocking the thinking processes). Initially the counsellor did not acknowledge the emotional state and the interactional sequence was repeated. However, as soon as the counsellor used empathy to connect with the patient, the interaction was unlocked and the interview changed.

Example

A woman consulted the genetic department as her husband and his brother had both died of a stroke. She wondered if the two deaths were the result of a genetic disorder. She was worried that her children were at risk and thought that they needed to be assessed and their health monitored. She had not been able to speak directly to the children and wanted the counsellor to tell her children 'a white lie', or any story, to engage them in a monitoring programme. She did not want them to know 'the truth' about what she thought was their genetic vulnerability.

The counsellor explained that, given the age of her husband and his brother, strokes were common problems and they were not likely to be genetically linked, but conceded that there could be renal problems, with associated high blood pressure. The woman repeatedly asked the same question about whether the counsellor would talk to her children. In reply the counsellor answered with an repeated educative interventions, trying harder and harder to explain the possible causes of strokes and the chances of there being a genetic element involved. The patient was unable to take in any information and kept returning to her own idea that if the doctor would tell the children 'a white lie', they would be looked after.

The woman's ability to take in information was blocked by her agitation. The counsellor then picked up the woman's remark of, 'It would be terrible to survive one's children, they've suffered enough' and responded with an emotional, not educative, intervention. 'You seem convinced that you are going to lose your children in the same way you lost your husband. You seem so frightened about that possibility that I can't reassure you that the likelihood is extremely rare. As you say, in losing their father they have indeed suffered and I can understand that you want to protect them'.

At that point the woman broke down and said that even though her husband had died 8 years ago, it seemed like yesterday. Movingly, the patient described the details of her husband's death, how the children were present and how she and her children had not spoken about it together. The counsellor then volunteered 'I wonder if the pain you want to protect your children from has actually happened. Your belief is that by not speaking about it helps, but I wonder whether they, like you, would be relieved to speak and share their grief'. The woman concluded, 'I've not known what to do for the best, it's really blown me apart . . . .'

Reflecting on this interview it can be seen that when the counsellor changed from a repeated educative intervention to an emotional one, the interview pattern changed. The intervention had a number of components; an understanding of the patient's fear and an acknowledgement of the desire and intent to protect her children from pain. It also included a comment on the interactional dynamic, which acknowledged the counsellor's failure to reassure. The woman's distress was then contained and, as a result, the consultation was refocussed and reframed as unresolved grief.

Acknowledging the woman's internally disrupted experiences gave her an opportunity of processing them in an empathic relationship. As a result they were thoughtfully digested and transformed.

Watzlawich et al. (1974) defined reframing as changing 'the conceptual and/or the emotional setting or viewpoint in relation to which a situation is experienced and to place it in another frame which fits the "facts" equally well or even better and thereby changes its entire meaning'. Asen and Jones (2000) consider that one of the intentions when reframing is to change from a frame which is unalterable to one that is implicitly flexible and open to change. The examples given in earlier chapters have used reframing when working with couples and put a positive construction on a difficulty that a couple are experiencing. For example, the different opinions of a couple have been described as the couple working together to ensure all aspects of the dilemma are covered – the same situation but with a different meaning.

Working with coping defences

The stress of genetic counselling can be a considerable challenge to individuals and have varying effects depending on the meaning of the event and the characteristics of the individual. Sometimes, this results in mental defence mechanisms being called upon to afford protection from reality and help the individual to cope. Occasionally, defences breakdown and the individual collapses, as is demonstrated in the first example. Individuals tend to have their own particular coping style which endures and, even within the same family, different members can react in different ways. With time, especially if there is a supportive relationship, the individual moves towards adjustment. In the next examples the individuals have made some adjustment but the counsellor's contribution facilitated the process further.

Describing and naming the process
Example

A woman consulted the genetic department after learning that her estranged mother was in hospital and was suffering from Huntington's disease. She described to the counsellor how, on hearing the news, she was devastated and fell apart. She could not work but stayed in bed all day crying. After a few days, she could begin to think about what she might do and decided she would seek information from the genetic department.

The counsellor responded by empathising with her on how upsetting it must have been to have such distressing news and went on to name her difficulty by commenting, 'You've obviously been shocked, frightened and been through a sort of grieving process. Your world was turned upside down and you lost how you thought things were. You didn't really know what to do initially and didn't know how to manage and in a grief state went to bed. Now, you are attempting to get yourself together again, you have worked through the shock and are adjusting. What's more you are addressing the problem and wanting to find out about yourself and whether you have the gene'.

The counsellor's intervention may seem very simple. However, it involved more than sympathising with her distress as, in addition, the counsellor named and described the emotional process the individual was going through as shock and grief. That demonstrated the counsellor had understood the upset, and the reason for it. Mirroring and making appropriate statements of understanding the upset can be helpful. However, to understand and explain that she had been struggling to cope with shock and grief and that she has been making an attempt to recover, provided a framework for thought. Labelling the process provides an understanding of the intent. It encapsulates the patient's whole process, integrating the emotional experience and the underlying process of resolution. Using the words shock, grief and adjustment gives the patient an anchor to tell herself what she has been through; telling her how well she has done and that she is beginning to master this difficulty. Most importantly by naming the process as adjustment, it allows the woman to think, 'I've been shocked, I'm upset, I'm adjusting', which is triggering a self-reflective state of mind.

Understanding and naming the process
Example

In this second example the stress response is different but the counsellor uses a similar intervention.

> Two sisters have different ways of trying to deal with their upset about learning that their father had died of Huntington's disease. The sisters consulted the department separately; the one came alone, the other with her mother. In the second interview with mother and daughter, the mother commented on the difference between her daughters. She described how, on hearing of the father's illness, one daughter had tried to read as much as she could to find about the disorder and had come for a consultation alone. In contrast, the other daughter had busied herself cleaning the house and wanted her mother to accompany her. The counsellor responded by speaking to the daughter and saying,
>
> 'You have been struggling with the shock of this news and when you first heard you didn't know what to do, but things have changed a little as now you are here'. The daughter replied:
>
> 'I just can't believe it, I have to keep doing things. I was planning to get married and now this, I'm so frightened I will lose my boy friend'.
>
> The counsellor asked about her relationship and found out that the boyfriend had been very supportive and so ventured the following idea, 'I wonder, if when you heard this news about your father, you were extremely shocked and it turned your life upside down. You believed you had lost everything, your own future health and your future marriage. Your way of dealing with all this has been to try to keep busy, trying to tidy everything up, as if too frightened to stop. But I guess you've found that the upset stays there'.

'That's right' the daughter replied, 'It's such a shock …'and she started to cry. 'I haven't cried since I was told, I was sort of stunned'. The counsellor replied,

'You seem to have moved a long way in adjusting to the news, you were initially quite shocked and then very distressed. I would guess you were frightened and grieving for the loss of your life as it was. And now you are here to talk about it all and find you can cry'. The woman responded:

'Yes, I want to know and stop imagining the worst all the time. Maybe I haven't got it but, if I have, my boy friend and I will have to talk and think'.

Both daughters were attempting to manage the pain, the one by intellectualisation and the other by displacement activity. The defence of intellectualisation brings people for a consultation, facilitates understanding and planning and gives a sense of control. However, displacement activity is an attempt to get control of what is experienced as uncontrollable feelings. In the woman's description it is possible to hear her shock at the news of her father's illness, and also that she is experiencing another stress as she feels her future marriage may be threatened. As in the last example the counsellor's intervention did not simply mirror her feelings, as it also gave the woman an understanding and explanation of her need for a defence. The processes of shock, grief and adjustment were named which is equivalent to including an understanding of the intent. In addition, the intervention allowed the counsellor to reframe her behaviour as an attempt to deal with the shock of her news. It is interesting that the woman was then able to face the grief she had been avoiding and, subsequently, that allowed her to think in a more balanced way. The relationship with the counsellor had contained the woman agitation, which allowed her to emotionally process her distress and facilitate her thinking.

Supporting attempts to cope
Example

In the following example the counsellor highlights the woman's courage and determination, describing it conceptually as coping. The woman knows she has done well, but having someone else describe her efforts positively lets her know someone is listening and gives it validation.

A young woman had been attempting to struggle with her blindness and in a genetic consultation she said, 'People are trying, but they are being too helpful and I want to say, I want to shout at them, "Look I haven't lost my sight yet, I can still see, I can understand.

Leave me alone. Stop panicking'. I've got to look after myself. I can't expect anyone else to look after me. It's just confidence. I've got just enough confidence to go on the bus and say to the driver, Where am I? What bus am I on? And I'm thinking if anybody's laughing, fair play, carry on … it doesn't bother me any more. It used to bother me, I used to be very stressed, but now I don't care'.

The counsellor responded, 'You are obviously a fighter and determined to adjust to manage in the world. It's a new world and you are trying to find your way again. It is hard going but, you are struggling to maintain your independence when your sight is fading and, you are standing strong when others are not respectful. What you are finding is that your confidence is growing with practice and that gives you more confidence'.

The counsellor had applauded her spirited approach to difficulties and reinforced her belief in her ability to cope. A similar opportunity of being supportive was afforded when the woman explained that she couldn't read well as a child and that she hadn't been helped by either her family or the school. She remembered asking her mother to help with her home work and she got shouted at, as she had been at school. 'My education wasn't good, I learned nothing. I didn't know my alphabet when I left school. I didn't know my address, I didn't know how to spell my name properly. . . . But now I am learning with my five year old daughter. When I was young I was never taught, so now I am teaching myself how to read, write, how to do things'. The counsellor responded by recognising her determination and ability to learn and cope with adversity and said, 'You certainly know how to master and overcome adversity. There's nothing much you won't have a jolly good go at with enormous courage and, as you know, your sight isn't going to improve. The way you've learnt to adjust and master difficulties is going to stand you in good stead for any future problem you may have in life'.

Conveying this understanding to the woman was powerfully affirming. She knew that she was succeeding but knowing through someone else observing and recognising her struggle was very affirming. The counsellor also slips in the need for her to be strong in the future as her sight would not improve. The counsellor supported the woman's effective coping and seeded the idea she will need her coping skills in the future.

Triggering coping in the face of hopelessness

There are very many disorders which have a chronically debilitating course, depriving the individual of normal functioning and leading to a life of physical handicap and pain. The emotional distress can be accentuated when there is full awareness of the difficulty, the limitations, losses and lack of cure or treatment. The inability to help is difficult for the health worker to accept since the whole of their *raison d'être* is to be able to contribute and make a difference. The counsellor may have the idea that there is nothing to offer in a situation which is hopeless and this can result in the counsellor withdrawing in embarrassment, becoming defensive or depressed. However, the skill needed in this area is the ability to tolerate the inactivity and hopelessness. Staying with the individual's pain can be an enormous gift of compassion. In the following example the counsellor has to face therapeutic impotence or helplessness, knowing there is nothing anyone can do to change an extremely distressing situation. It is not easy to stay with someone in the terminal stages. This example demonstrates the importance of entering the patient's hopelessness so, paradoxically, becoming therapeutically potent in what initially appeared to be a hopeless situation.

Example

A couple asked for an appointment as they were finding it very difficult to cope as the wife had a severe form of Ehlers–Danlos syndrome which had led to her becoming extremely handicapped. Her joints needed to be splinted and supported by numerous cuffs, protecting them from any injury. She had suffered a number of episodes of bleeding into many organs and knew her life was on a knife-edge. Both partners were extremely angry and upset. They told the counsellor how much they had lost: her health, their life together, their ability to have fun, their future. They had no children and had no hope of any. For her, the loss of her working position equated with a loss of her role in society and as a contributor in the home – a sort of loss of identity. For him, the loss of future children was hardest to bear. He had also given up his job to be the carer. They were cut off from life and from one another by their individual despair; both of them had become isolated in her illness. Even everyday life was 'on hold'. The counsellor had an idea that they were paralysed by their rage and were, metaphorically, staring into space. Tentatively the counsellor asked about their anger and both acknowledged and expressed their fury.

This interview was very upsetting for the couple and for the counsellor. Witnessing such physical and emotional pain, anguish and isolation was challenging for the counsellor. It was important to be able to feel and tolerate the upset and yet not be personally too upset. The counsellor listened to their story of their different losses and how their lives had just fallen apart, leaving them both feeling cheated and extremely angry. The counsellor understood their anger but reframed it as helping them get rid of some of their awfulness and protecting them from becoming even more upset. The anger was labelled as a reaction to loss and a defence against too much loss.

About half way through the planned time, the counsellor changed the focus to the sadness of them not having any hope and it not being possible for the counsellor to be able to offer any hope of physical improvement. The counsellor said: 'The worst thing for you is that there is nothing you can do and nothing anyone can do. I too feel sad I can't do anything to change things for you'. The counsellor took the risk of asking, 'So I'm wondering how you are going to live in the middle of all this?'

This was followed by an exploration of how each had coped with adversity in the past and of people they had known who had found a way of living in the middle of enormous difficulties. They both engaged in this investigation, exploring their resources, previous adjustments and coping experiences. It included wondering how they could have some pleasant moments in the day, or what might comfort them.

Finally, towards the end of the session when the mood was lighter, their problems were likened to being attacked by a storm which was hitting them from all sides. This metaphor seemed to have particular meaning for the woman who said, 'I'm almost ship-wrecked, but not completely, so it's really a matter of finding the quiet centre in the middle of the storm', and the counsellor agreed.

This interview is an example of the counsellor staying with the awfulness, acknowledging the distress, but, not being overwhelmed by it. Accompanying the woman through her storm allowed her to find her quiet centre. The challenge, put out by the counsellor, of asking how she was going to live in the middle of the distress could have been extremely aggressive. However, the counsellor had earned a position of trust through tolerating the considerable upset earlier in the interview. In taking the freedom to challenge, the counsellor facilitated freedom in the patient and turned a sense of hopeless into an exploration of internal resources.

Working with attachment patterns and defences

In his paper 'Relatively speaking': relativisation of genetic risk in counselling for predictive testing, Sarangi et al. (2003) point out how, in any one interview, the counsellor attempts to give the patient a realistic view of risk by generalising or giving statistics. However, where the patient is distorting the information the counsellor may have to use strategies, which sometimes escalate and sometimes de-escalate the risk, depending on the way the individual perceives the facts. So for those individuals who are minimising the risk, the counsellor may have to emphasise reality and, conversely, where the individual has an exaggerated view, the counsellor may need to correct the misperception by de-escalating. Sarangi et al. are commenting on how the counsellor changes style to counter the distortions, brought about by the defensive style of the patient.

In the following example a counsellor is faced with a couple who are not able to enter the spirit of talking and thinking about themselves. They use a dismissive attachment pattern and block all discussion about testing for Huntington's disease.

Example

A couple requested a consultation as the woman has a family history of Huntington's disease. Both her parents had died when she was a child and she had been brought up by foster parents. She had been told as a teenager that her father had died from Huntington's disease and that she should have a test before having any children. She now has a partner and they want a child but, she was very clear that she would not have a child if she had the Huntington's disease gene. She stated very clearly she wanted to be tested. The counsellor found it extremely difficult to open up any discussion and felt it was impossible to make any contact with either of the couple. They were in total agreement, there was no exploration or debate, every thought introduced by the counsellor was blocked and the couple repeatedly expressed their desire for the test.

Such a situation is extremely worrying as it begs the question of whether the couple are fully aware of the consequences of testing and whether they have any flexibility in their thinking. Their emotional repertoire was equally restricted, with no sign of affection between them. In addition, the counsellor was unable to establish any emotional rapport and was left feeling shut out and de-skilled, with the tools of empathy and understanding being of little use.

Using attachment theory the couple could both be seen as having an insecure pattern, with all pain and exploration dismissed. The most likely hypothesis would be that the woman's early emotional pain and possible deprivation had been very traumatic and was reflected not only in personal style of managing stress, but also in the lack of emotion in the couple's relationship.

The genetic counsellor tried a number of different strategies under the extremely difficult circumstances.

1. The use of explanations and explorations

The counsellor began by explaining that the idea of the discussion was not to put obstacles in their way to prevent them having the test but was designed to help them understand the importance of the decision and the consequences. This was followed by an invitation for them to explore in imagination their responses to possible different test results. They did not engage in the exercise and repeated their request to be tested.

2. The use of empathy

The counsellor made an empathic comment about the difficulty of the discussion and speculated that it might be frightening. This was ignored and, trying again, the counsellor ventured that some people just grit their teeth when they are frightened and tell themselves they just need to get on with it. Neither of these strategies resulted in opening up a discussion.

3. Commenting on the interactional dynamic and declaring a personal difficulty

The counsellor ventured the following intervention, 'I'm feeling a bit stuck, we don't seem to be able to switch into one another's wave length. We seem to be thinking differently, I'm trying to invite you to take your time in your decision to be tested, to pause a moment and consider what it might be like to have a result of carrying the gene. You however, are quite certain you want the test and I understand that you need to know before embarking on a pregnancy. My experience is such that you may find it helpful to explore your feelings a little. I wonder whether either of you is in any way worried?' The response was again blank looks.

The worry when an interview is so closed and sterile is that the rather rigid defence used by the individual will break down and uncover a seriously fragmented inner world. In addition, the counsellor can become frustrated by the lack of discussion. At the end of a rather unsatisfactory meeting the couple were invited to attend for their second appointment. In that consultation, the woman revealed that she was pregnant and that they did not want to have the test. The counsellor was very surprised and refrained from commenting on their earlier statement of not having children if the woman did carry the Huntington's disease gene.

It was puzzling that the woman had stated very clearly she would not have a child if she tested positive, yet, in a short space of time, she had become pregnant. Several questions remain unanswered but, most importantly, when did the woman know she was pregnant? Was she pregnant at the time of the initial consultation or had she become pregnant in the intervening time? If the former were true, it could explain the complete blocking of all the counsellor's best efforts in the original meeting. The latter could be explained by unconscious desires over-riding her more logical self. The couple offered no explanations leaving the counsellor feeling depressed and feeling something had been missed.

In conclusion, this chapter has offered the genetic counsellor some clinical examples to demonstrate the use of the ideas put forward in the earlier chapters. The stories are different but have the common theme of the counsellor's empathy being the effective common denominator.

The gene and the family system

The counsellor frequently has a family group in the consultation, a nuclear family, an extended family or multigenerational. The counsellor's practice will be enhanced by an understanding of how 'the group' is a unit to be thought of as a whole, yet made up of interacting parts. This chapter presents the core features of systemic thinking and its application to genetic counselling. It integrates this way of thinking with that of the earlier chapters, in particular attachment theory, in order to provide a consistent theoretical base for working in genetic counselling.

The clinical practice of genetic counselling includes in its orbit the psychosocial context of the family history of relationships and looks at how individual members of a family interact together and mutually affect one another. It looks at the communication patterns of particular members of a family, their emotional links and how the story of the gene is spoken about in the family life cycle. This immediately introduces systemic thinking, yet with notable exceptions (Eunpu, 1997), it has not been widely used in genetic counselling. Indeed some counsellors are rather intimidated by systemic theory which can at times be complicated and philosophical in its discussions and seem far removed from the distressing problems experienced by families.

Thinking systemically

Systemic thinking is a way of viewing the world based on an understanding of the natural system of the world, the way it is held in balance, the interdependence of its parts and the far reaching effect of change in any one part (Bateson, 1973). Consequently, everything can be viewed from a systemic perspective and everything is in an environmental context. For example, the gene is part of the body system and a change in a gene, one part of the body system, will effect changes in other parts of the body system and, with or without other factors, the potential for disease is released. Genetic counselling includes the study of the social aspects around the gene in the context the social system of family relationships, beliefs and relationship patterns across generations.

An understanding of general principles of systemic theory and its application to families in genetic counselling is presented to demonstrate its importance in enriching clinical practice.

Characteristics of a system, the family system, subsystems and the consultation system

Street (1994) identifies the characteristics of a naturally occurring system as being composed of inter-related parts which combine to influence its total functioning where the patterns of connection are established by information from one part to the other. The boundary around the system is arbitrary and the balance within is maintained by a process of feedback. The word 'system' can be used to describe any group of people where they are interacting with one another. In the family system the interactions are relatively stable and recursive and form the context for individual development, functioning and satisfaction. Any system will change to become a new system with the addition or removal of members. As a result, a system cannot be observed, as the addition of 'the observer' creates a new system. In practice this means once the counsellor comes into the family system, a new system develops – that of 'the family and the counsellor'. It becomes the consultation system, indicating that the boundary around the family, or any other system, is open and flexible allowing movement in and out.

The family is a social system made up of a group of individuals of different generations that interact with one another over time. In genetic counselling it is usually considered over three generations. Within the family system there will be subsystems such as the parental system made up of the parents and a child system constituted by the children. Individual members of a family will belong to other groups and, in a similar way, the genetic counsellor is part of other groups. In particular, the counsellor belongs to a professional system. All of these other systems impinge and have an influence on the consultation system.

The family system is the cultural context within which genetic information is handled and contains attitudes and beliefs about the genetic disorder and, most importantly, it is the context within which decisions are made (Soldan et al., 2000). The counsellor knows from clinical experience that the system is more than a sum of its parts and has a quality of wholeness so that every family has its own identity and can be recognised by its characteristic interactional style (Jones, 1993). Each family will have its own distinctive communication pattern which is influenced by past and present members, with specifies attitudes, beliefs, relationships and, in particular, the organisation of intimacy (Evans and Street, 2003).

Thinking systemically with an individual

It might appear that the genetic counsellor either works individually or systemically depending on whether an individual or a family is in the consulting room. Although the counsellor might work differently under those circumstances, in reality the consultation is always systemic. In an individual consultation, the counsellor and individual make up the consultation system, but the family is always in the room. It is not actually present, but alive within the individual influencing thinking and behaviour. The individual carries the family history and experience of being in it as a memory in the mind. It influences the individual attitudes and pattern of relating to the world. It is also in the individual's body, as a physical memory and expression of history. In addition the counsellor is also part of professional and personal systems which influence thinking and attitudes resulting in a number of ideas from other systems impinging on the consultation system.

The genetic counsellor, knowingly or unknowingly, is a systemic thinker as working in genetics makes that inevitable. For instance, the counsellor is using systemic thinking when exploring how the individual has been influenced by past family relationship patterns and communication styles which contain family beliefs and attitudes. In addition, an individual is considered in the context of the present family system and the counsellor wonders how any new information will affect other members, as well as how they are affecting the individual concerned.

Example

A 16-year-old girl asked to be seen as she wanted to be tested for Huntington's disease. She revealed that several members of her mother's family had the disorder and she wanted to know her own genetic status. In exploring the history of the disorder in the family and how she became aware of it, she revealed her worries that her mother had refused testing and would not speak about her family.

The counsellor's assessment was that the young girl appeared to have a good grasp of the issues and she seemed more mature than her chronological age. However, if she were to be tested and found to have the mutation she would be carrying information for a long time and, in addition, it would have implications for her mother. The daughter understood the complexity and agreed to the counsellor contacting the parents to discuss the problem.

In that meeting the counsellor was surprised that not only did the mother have symptoms, but that they were quite marked and obvious. The counsellor began by explaining that she had come because their daughter was requesting testing and the marital couple acknowledged that they knew of their daughter's request. It was explained that testing the daughter could change things for them in possibly confirming the mother's status. The couple understood and acknowledged that there had always been a difference of opinion between them; the husband wanting his wife to be tested, the wife preferring not to know. Further, they did not feel that they would change their minds. Whilst it was not acknowledged that the woman was symptomatic, the counsellor felt that the couple knew but did not want it named. They had obviously decided that their way of dealing with the dilemma was to not face it.

With this added information the girl's request for a consultation could then be reconsidered in the context of a mother who had symptoms and a family culture of not acknowledging the obvious. The information introduced various hypotheses about the meaning of the daughter's request to be tested. Did the daughter want an answer to her request for testing, or was she saying 'Come and help me with my parents?' She could also have been saying 'Come and help my parents' or 'Come and talk to my family as we are not talking about the obvious difficulty'.

The daughter did not continue with her request and again various hypotheses came to mind. Had the daughter's mission been achieved by introducing another person who could facilitate a conversation which otherwise could not take place within the family? Alternatively, how could she proceed with testing? She had heard her parents say the situation would not change and she knew that if tested she might have information which would demolish her mother's denial. She could of course have decided to wait, knowing that change would be inevitable for her mother and that she could be tested in the future. She may have concluded that, for the moment, the problem could be solved by her agreeing with the family pattern of self-protection.

In this individual consultation the counsellor had considered the systemic effect of testing the girl and the implications for the mother. As a consequence, after visiting the family, the meaning of the girl's request could be reformulated in the context of the family denial.

The attachment dynamic and systemic thinking

Attachment theory and systemic thinking are two major philosophical frameworks which direct the counsellor's behaviour. It would be important to realise that the theories do not conflict such that they need to be separated with the one used when working with an individual and the other when working with families. Attachments are the bedrock of families and determine how a family negotiates closeness and distance, emotional containment, conflict and autonomy and will affect how the genetic inheritance is dealt with.

A number of psychotherapeutic thinkers have explored the integration of systemic and attachment ideas. Heard (1982) achieved this by introducing the concept of the attachment dynamic. She considered it provided an explanation of how individual members of a family behave as though they constituted a system and the extent to which the family had complimentary care-giving behaviour. The dynamic was considered to govern the movements of family members towards and away from one another. It affected the degree to which they engaged in exploratory activities and influenced the internal representation each member built of him- or herself in relation to others or acting alone. Put more simply, Heard considered the way individuals were attached to care for one another made up the family system and its nature determined whether they were could be close and could explore the world.

Kozlowska and Hanney (2002) considered that attachment and family systems theory have shared common origins in moving away from psychoanalysis towards an emphasis on real relationships. They discussed the integration of the theories and proposed 'network thinking' which requires the clinician to hold multiple perspectives in mind, moving from one to the other as necessary. This avoids the debate about the distinct nature of these theories and the possibility of them being integrated. It proposes looking at levels of complexity of the dyad and family as distinct, yet interconnected.

Park (2004) proposed another idea of treating each major theoretical school as if it were a language and develops the idea of being multilingual (whilst not forgetting the mother tongue).

There is no attachment school of family therapy, but Byng-Hall (1995b) has been a major influence in using attachment theory in thinking about families. He defined a secure family base as 'a family that provides a reliable network of attachment relationships which enables the family members of whatever age to feel sufficiently secure to explore relationships with each other and with others outside the family'. He goes on to explain that the family understands that attachment relationships need to be protected and not undermined and that support for one another is paramount. He believes the motto of the secure family is 'collaborate to care'.

Securely attached families are able to be flexible, supporting one another through challenging situations with individuals moving closer together at times of stress, but not impinging too much on each other. Most importantly, in securely attached families emotions can be processed so that grief can be managed and anxiety contained. With insecure attachment patterns, the situation is different. At the dismissive end of the spectrum the needs of individuals are not met and the importance of the emotional significance is minimised; whereas at the preoccupied end of the attachment spectrum, people are trapped in over-involvement, impingement and heightened emotions which are not contained or processed.

Whilst being relatively stable over time, the family also needs to be change to allow for developmental progress and crisis situations. Families differ in their degree of flexibility (Olsen et al., 1988) and that will determine the ability to cope with change. Folkman (1984) has categorised the resources needed by the family under three headings: material (relating to the economic resources), physical (which are to do with health and fitness) and social (to include practical and emotional support within the family and wider system). The task for the family is how to collaborate to manage stress, conflict, share emotions and support one another.

Family themes and stresses and the idea of the gene as another element

Byng-Hall (1995a, p. 106) considers that the situations which undermine the capacity for the family to provide a secure base include: fear of losing or actual loss of an attachment figure, unusually strong and inappropriate pairings, conflict within relationships and expectation of repetition of losses similar to those encountered in previous generations.

The central pairing in any family is the parental couple and the quality of that relationship is a key factor in the family security. Conflict or deficiencies in that relationship can leave all family members feeling insecure. Actual loss of a parent is traumatic but can be managed with the support from another important figure. The threat of loss through repeated rows or separations can be as destabilising as actual loss. Sometimes the deficiencies in the couple relationship draw in and inappropriately involve one of the children who then becomes an adult's confidante. That process is called triangulation and the family is then skewed and results in it providing insecure attachment experiences. Clearly, chronic illness frequently leads to loss or fear of loss and, in addition, triggers further challenges by necessitating a change in family roles. These can result in the child becoming a carer for an adult in the family creating what is called a 'parentified child' who has to behave like a responsible adult, whilst not being appropriately mature.

Information about a genetic disorder could be thought of as another element which needs to be included in the family system. It requires the family to adjust to the 'new arrival', in the same way as a birth or death triggers an adjustment relating to the life cycle. The family has to find a new perception of itself whether it is as a result of genetic information or a life cycle change. New knowledge interferes with the family sense of control and challenges the degree of intimacy with the family needing to create new relationship patterns to address issues of inclusion, control and intimacy.

The family attachment experiences will determine the degree of flexibility and resourcefulness and result in either adaptation or the creation of defensive measures to avoid the painful issue. Most families find their way through the new genetic knowledge but, in some, it can be the axis around which relationship difficulties are acted out. Flexible families are capable of re-organisation and change, but if the interactional pattern is too rigid, then the family will become 'stuck' and difficulties arise. It is at this point that, in less flexible families, secrets arise, or relationships are strained or broken, with blame or shame colouring the scene. From a systemic point of view, the questions are how does the family re-organise itself around its new knowledge and, what adjustments have to be made for the family to find a new balance? Genetic knowledge becomes an element added to the family belief about itself and the new system is the family plus the idea of the gene.

In the following example a couple are unable to cope with the potential of new genetic information directly. Their family stability, previously found in denial is put under threat by a pregnancy.

Example

A couple requested a consultation to discuss the genetic status of their unborn child. The father had a family history of Huntington's disease and adamantly rejected any thought of being tested himself. In the interview the couple were given appropriate information and helped to think through testing the foetus and the implications for the father and the child. They remained as they were at the beginning of the interview – seeking testing of the foetus. They hoped to avoid personal knowledge and were gambling on the fact that his unborn child would not have the gene (which would allow him to continue in uncertainty). When asked how they would use the information from the testing of the foetus, they again revealed their difficulties by saying they did not know.

Before the pregnancy, the family culture had been one of avoiding knowledge of personal genetic status, excluding the idea and attempting to maintain a sense of sameness through avoidance. However, the conception of a child and the possibility that it could be affected had destabilised the couple, triggering anxiety at the threat of potential change.

This scenario presents the counsellor with a dilemma. The counsellor's task could be seen as informing the couple of the consequences of testing the foetus to include the implications for the father. With the counsellor's responsibility discharged, they could be left alone to make their own decision. However, the counsellor had two main concerns: one of depriving the unborn child of the right to personal choice in an adult-onset disease; the other, of clarifying whether the couple were emotionally prepared for a test result. The result of testing the foetus could leave the father in his 'not-knowing' position. Equally, it could confirm him as possessing the Huntington's genetic mutation. The man's avoidance of direct testing of himself suggested he had difficulty confronting his own vulnerability, both genetically and psychologically. To date, he had avoided the potential for grief associated with information and sought confirmation of his hope that his child would not be carrying the gene. The counsellor's assessment was that he had an insecure attachment pattern and needed the defence of denial and avoidance to protect him. The concern would be that these patterns would not serve him well in coping with a change in his genetic status.

It can be very frustrating for the counsellor to be faced with rigid defences which block open conversation. The counsellor may feel locked out, rendered useless and at risk of acting out the frustration by becoming agitated or impatient.

The counsellor would probably attempt a number of several strategies to help the couple. One intervention would be an educative approach, dealing with the consequences of testing the foetus; in contrast, the second would be emotional. The latter would involve a sensitive enquiry about the man's knowledge and experience of the condition in his family, which would include family patterns of dealing with the disorder. That discussion might reveal his fears and also afford the counsellor an opportunity to empathically support him. It would involve inviting him to explore how it might be if the foetus tested positively for the gene, how that would affect him, his relationship with his partner and their attitude to the foetus. Similar questions would also be directed to the wife to understand her thinking. Throughout this sensitive consultation the counsellor would be attempting to provide a secure base for the couple to think and feel their way through the highly charged situation.

Using a different approach, the counsellor could empathically state that they have obviously struggled with this dilemma before coming and then to ask – 'What sort of discussions have you had?' or 'How hard has it been to come to your agreement?' These questions do not ask 'Have you discussed this?' and 'Did you find it hard?' Rather, there is an assumption that the situation is difficult, the exploration is therefore about their dynamic around the decision, rather than a challenge to the decision itself. It avoids directly focusing on their conclusion, rather, moves out from that to them and their relationship. Further questions might be, 'Which of you will be most upset if your baby tests positively?' and 'How will you comfort one another?' These questions look for difference and discussion (as well as stating that there will be upset) rather than asking 'Will you be upset?' They invite the couple to think about comfort and support and their patterns of sharing distress.

Family roles and scripts and preselection

In their functioning, families unconsciously agree and allot roles to their members, such as 'the organiser', 'the comforter' and so on. Kessler (1988) has described a process in Huntington's disease which he has termed preselection, whereby a child is singled out as the one who will eventually develop the condition. He describes how the preselection occurs when the parent first begins to show symptoms – the function of the process being to protect other members from anxiety. Particular similar characteristics are identified linking the selected child to the affected parent and generalised to include having Huntington's disease. This has a profound affect on the selected individual who speaks of when, not if, they will develop the condition (Richards, 1996). Sometimes, however, the selected person may not be aware of what is being done. In an earlier chapter on attachment an example is given of the devastation a man experiences when the preselection process adopted by the family does not concur with the reality of testing.

Preselection is a particular form of what family therapists call family scripts (Byng-Hall, 1995b) which refer to the beliefs and stories a family constructs about family relations. In genetic counselling, the scripts will be built around the meaning and interpretation the family have given to their family history and how the problem has arisen. The family tree is a useful format for their exploration. Where an abnormality appears *de novo*, the family has to construct a narrative to understand the event. This narrative may include elements of folklore or superstitions which are used to give meaning to chance happenings or illnesses. Part of the task of a genetic consultation is to facilitate the development by the family of a story which incorporates the genetic information. This might mean that an individual's original script may need to be changed to include accurate information about genetic inheritance patterns and a test result. The family security and flexibility will determine whether the new genetic information can be incorporated to develop a new story.

The family tree

The genetic consultation makes use of the family genogram (McGoldrick and Gerson, 1985) which diagrammatically maps the path of the gene across the generations. The consultation is both a factual genetic history and a social interactional history. The process of drawing up a family tree in genetic counselling can have profound effects on family relationships (Richards, 1996). Memories of births, deaths and illnesses are needed. It may mean searching for information from other family members so challenging the relationships, or renewing contact with an estranged member. The consultation is often the trigger for opening the family chest and uncovering its secrets. The emotional hurt and trauma of severed or strained relationships emerge and, in particular, experiences around the genetic illness are brought to the surface. Every individual is loaded with a history and when a genetic consultation creates a psychological space it affords an opportunity to metaphorically put the load down by talking about what, for some, is a very painful subject.

Family communication

The family communicative pattern will reveal how they deal with upset and challenge, which will include their management of closeness and distance. It will clarify their style of dismissal or exaggeration of events and feelings. An important factor contributing to a healthy adaptation is whether the genetic inheritance can be spoken about or whether it is too awful to name. The following example is of a family where the minimum is said about the genetic disorder, but a lot is understood.

Example

The counsellor asked a patient, 'Is it something that you talk about in the family, quite a bit or not so much?' The reply was 'When I first used to come down here – well just before I first came down – anyway, they told me a few things but before they kept it all quiet. I don't think they wanted anyone to know. But my mother, well, she talks a bit more now … But my mother will say things now like 'I'm going to see the doctor'. I think the last time she came down with my auntie … She tells me stuff like that now, but before I came to see you and before I said about it, or whatever, she was, well, she didn't say anything like that. . . . You know, she wouldn't say anything. But I ask her and she will say stuff now'.

In this extract from a consultation, the patient has described the way she has understood the family pattern of dealing with its family history. She has made it clear that the subject of their genetic problem is difficult for the family to openly acknowledge. However, there is an understanding that although the messages are coded and indirect, the problem is half-acknowledged. So words such as 'going to see the doctor' mean that there is a genetic problem and it requires monitoring. This family have found a way of understanding their communication pattern. In some families, there is total embargo on any discussion of the problem and under those circumstances the embargo can carry an added valency which attracts dread, secrets or relationship difficulties.

Who attends the consultation?

The counsellor learns a considerable amount about the intergenerational relationship patterns by observing the composition of the group attending for a consultation. The composition tells a story. In a similar way, a lot can be learnt about the dynamics of the group by observing the selection of the spokesperson and the reaction of the other members. In particular, who is silent, who is upset or who is performing particular roles (comforter, peacemaker or challenger). The counsellor will need to be aware of everyone in the consultation, their behaviour, emotional expression and role. The counsellor might begin by asking, 'How did you decide to come today?' and 'Who was most interested in coming?' Or 'Who least wanted to come?' to give an idea of the motivation for the consultation. A question such as, 'Who would like to tell me something about the family history?' reveals the spokesperson of the family. The systemic thinker takes this further and asks the opinions of others in the interview by asking, 'Is that how you see it, or would you tell a slightly different story?' Another interesting question especially if there are children present would be, 'Is this the first time you've heard this story, or did you know it already', and further 'How did you learn about this story?' so looking at communication across the generations.

If the counsellor has a hypothesis that the family has difficulties in emotional expression then the question could be asked, 'I'm wondering how you deal with upset?' or 'Who gets upset and who comforts in your family?' and possibly following by tracking the sequence by, 'And what happens when you get upset?' All these questions are useful, not only in a factual sense, but they also allow an exploration of how the individuals behave together. The counsellor might take this further by asking 'Would you like things to be different?', or 'If X behaved in this way how would that affect you?' and 'Would that be better or worse?' With this questioning the counsellor is inviting an exploration of different behaviours and how that would systemically ripple through out the family. The counsellor asks questions which look at family interactional patterns to stimulate thinking about how the family is interconnected as this reflective way of thinking can facilitate change (Street,

1994). The counsellor offers an opportunity to experience different ways of dealing with problems and their emotional consequences.

The questions which have been proposed are examples of what family therapists call 'circular interviewing'. The interviewing technique follows a circular or spiralling pattern where the feedback to the counsellor's question shapes the next question and so on. The counsellor is then both conducting the interview and responding to the family. It is perhaps important to point out that the technique applies to the conversation between counsellor and individual as it does to the interaction between counsellor and family.

'Circular interviewing' involves a particular interest in questions of *difference* as in difference there is identity and clarification (Asen and Jones, 2000). For example, 'Are you more or less anxious?' 'Has it brought you closer or more distant from your sister?' Questions are constructed that look at difference over time, frequently around a particular point in time. For example, 'How have you been since you had your test result?' The questions may look at ranking – 'Who will be most upset by this news?' Triadic questions invite one person to comment on their perception of an aspect of the relationship between two other individuals. For example, 'Help me understand how your mother and father are working out their ideas about how much to tell the rest of the family'. The function of all these questions is to reveal the family interactional dynamic around the issue or dilemma – helping the family think self-reflectively.

The tasks of the counsellor when working with a family

At the beginning of the clinical encounter with a family the counsellor takes the family history and constructs a family tree. This provides information about the family interactional pattern and their relationship with the counsellor. In particular, the counsellor will be assessing the family's ability to collaborate to manage stress and the degree to which conflict interrupts its adaptive functioning. This clarifies the nature of the family attachment pattern and whether the family can act as a secure-enough base for one another to help in the challenge of genetic counselling. The families with an insecure attachment pattern will need more help from a counsellor than a family with a secure pattern. Families with a secure attachment patterns are able to express, share and contain emotions, in preparation for decision-making or a test result. The stress of genetic counselling can be particularly challenging and even securely attached families frequently need counselling help. The task of the counsellor is to provide a secure-enough base for the family to discuss and think about its genetic inheritance. In working with families the counsellor will be attempting to attune to all members of the family (not just that of one individual) in order to understand their different perspectives. In addition, the counsellor empathically relates to the family as a whole, to understand the way they all link together to form a pattern of relationships. The counsellor's availability to all the members of the family creates a secure-enough base in the consultation to facilitate an open discussion around the genetic issues. In insecurely attached families the counsellor's principal task will be to help in the particular problem area. Strategies which help support problem-solving include the resolution of conflict and support of the central couple relationship (Byng-Hall, 1995a, p. 75). Those factors would be important in genetic counselling but, in addition, the counsellor may need to facilitate the containment of emotions and help the family work with their defences, to enable the family to make a decision and cope with a test result. The empathic availability of the counsellor to all members is the central factor determining the success of the consultation. The importance of the therapist's warmth in establishing a good working or therapeutic alliance and the importance of the three inter-related components of goal setting, tasks and a strong affective bond (Bordin, 1982) has already been discussed. These are equally valid in working with couples or families.

There may be two counsellors in a family consultation and their interaction together gives important messages to the family. They may choose to speak together within a consultation demonstrating open discussion and may even disagree as long as the disagreement is discussed. Such an experience would act as a model for the family confirming that conflict can be resolved. The principles of warmth and respect between the two professionals can influence a consultation as their relationship also acts as a model of openness for the family. The counsellors may be from different specialities or different professions bringing different skills. Clarification of the purpose of consultation and the different roles of the counsellors is the prerequisite to understanding how each behaves in the consultation. These roles can be explained to the family at the beginning of the consultation.

Attachment and detachment in family development and autonomy and life cycle

The parent/child attachment changes over time to allow for the developing independence in the child. The degree of detachment increases until the child reaches the stage of an autonomous adult. The attachment and detachment process is a dynamic involving the child moving away from the parent and the parent letting go the child. Through out this period the child develops other attachments outside the family and in adulthood finds a sexual partner to establish another family. These changes in the family are part of the family life cycle which has particular transition points of change – birth, infancy, childhood, adolescence, adulthood, middle age, retirement and aging and death. These transition points are times of stress for the family as the change is negotiated.

It is not unusual for an intergenerational group to attend a consultation. This could mean a number of things: it demonstrates the supportive links across the family, acknowledges the intergenerational nature of the genetic problem, illustrates that the family has not established a clear boundary of differentiation across the generations. The latter situation is not uncommon in certain parts of this and other countries, creating an enmeshed family, where individual separation and autonomy are compromised for the sake of togetherness. This can pose a problem as it may interfere with the ability to find an intimate relationship with a partner. More importantly for genetic counselling, relationships which are too close do not provide a secure-enough bedrock for emotions to be processed, or conflict resolved. Relationships which are too close very often create situations where emotions run very high and thinking is compromised as a result.

The following example presents a mother and daughter coming together for a consultation. The behaviour of the counsellor is interesting as a psychological intervention is made to facilitate the consideration of the genetic aspects of the consultation.

Example

A young woman, who was well known to the genetic department, attended for early prenatal testing of her fifth pregnancy. She had one daughter, her son had died at the age of three from a degenerative condition, she had terminated one affected pregnancy and suffered an intra-uterine death of another. As on previous occasions, she attended with her mother and the same relationship pattern emerged. She repeatedly deferred to her mother, inviting her to think and speak for her.

Sadly, the prenatal testing confirmed another affected foetus. The young woman was devastated and cried that she could not go through another termination. Her mother, who was also very distressed, movingly volunteered that she would help look after the baby. However, the mother's support failed to comfort the daughter who seemed over-whelmed by her distress.

There were two counsellors in the consultation and one suggested that perhaps both the mother and daughter might like to talk on their own to one of the counsellors. In their discussion before the consultation the team had commented to one another on the absence of the woman's partner in previous consultations and acknowledged their own frustrations at the relationship between the mother and daughter.

In her individual consultation the daughter seemed to find her way through her con-fusion and distress and, without her mother offering to help, she was able to say she did want a termination.

In an equally distressing individual session with the other counsellor, the mother spoke of her guilt as she felt responsible for her daughter's dead babies. She explained that her guilt tied her to her daughter and that it differentiated her from the rest of the family. She spoke of her pain at the loss of her grandchildren and her wish to protect her daughter. As she got more upset, she revealed that when her daughter had been con-ceived, she had been having an affair. It had left her feeling guilty and, further, she believed that this was her punishment for the betrayal of her husband. She could accept punishment directed at her alone, but the fact that her daughter had to suffer in this way, seemed very cruel. As a result, she treated her daughter differently from the rest of the family, wanting to protect her and carry what she considered was her burden. The coun-sellor was able to empathise with the mother's emotional pain, allowing her to talk about her guilt, how that had affected her relationship with her daughter and had resulted in them staying close together. The consultation continued with the counsellor helping the woman process her grief but an educative intervention was also necessary to address the misunderstanding about her daughter's genetic difficulty.

From a counselling perspective the behaviour of the counsellors is particu-larly interesting. They chose to separate the mother and daughter. They made a psychological intervention introducing a developmental shift in the family dynamics which affirmed the daughter's autonomy. It is interesting that this psychological intervention enabled the genetic aspect of the inter-view to be concluded. As a result both women responded by thinking and speaking more freely. The daughter was enabled to think and reach a decision about her dilemma; the mother took the opportunity to speak about her guilt for the first time. This bold intervention was a creative move introducing more separation, supporting the natural patterns of family development for the purpose of individual thinking. The motive justified the action and was validated by the result. The seeds of the intervention can be found in the counsellors' thoughtful exploration of their own frustration, which had not been acted out, but constructively turned into an intervention.

A considerable amount of the genetic counsellor's work is not purely genetic as frequently it includes psychological work which has to be done to facilitate decision-making or coping with a test result. In addition, this example demonstrates the therapeutic potential in genetic counselling for a family's psychological growth.

The effect of a test result on a couple's relationship

Tibben (1993) have commented that in Huntington's disease it is the relationship, rather than the individual, which is most affected by the test result. In the next example the presenting problem is a deterioration in the couple relationship alongside the gene-carrier becoming depressed.

Example

A 35-year-old man requested testing as his father, one sister and brother were all affected by Huntington's disease. He agreed to the usual protocol of genetic counselling for presymptomatic testing and both he and his wife attended for a series of counselling consultations.

He began by giving the history of his father's erratic behaviour, alcohol abuse and ill treatment of the six children. The family of origin had not discussed the subject of Huntington's disease and, much to his wife's dismay, this pattern of not speaking was one of her husband's characteristics and had always been a problem in the marriage. Gene testing proved positive and the patient accepted it calmly saying it was what he had expected. He was reluctant to discuss this further and explained he just wanted to get on with his work.

Some time later his wife asked for a consultation as her husband had become very depressed and seemed to be experiencing a lot of difficulties. He had recently discovered that another brother had been tested for Huntington's disease and given a negative result and since then he had been unable to speak to his brother.

The couple were seen together and his wife tearfully spoke about the way she felt isolated and lonely as a result of her husband's withdrawal. Whereas she knew her husband had never wanted to discuss or share feelings, she now felt that since his result he had removed himself further. She then explained about his brother's result and how that seemed to make her husband even more depressed. Using a technique frequently used in family therapy, the counsellor asked the husband, 'Is that how you see it, is your wife's description a fair one, or do you see it differently?' (The technique involves seeking different viewpoints and examining interactional sequences of behaviour.) The husband acknowledged his habitual pattern of not communicating well and agreed that he had withdrawn more than usual, but concluded that was how he was. He explained that if he became upset he just worked it off. The counsellor ventured, 'I wonder if you are telling me that you have dealt with upset by sort of withdrawing into yourself and, until now, that has worked but, recently, it has not worked so well. Your long-standing pattern of working very hard physically is no longer effective'. He agreed and volunteered that he now could not sleep and working hard did not help any more. He just wanted to be left alone but his wife would not allow that and she kept shouting at him to talk. He had found that he was becoming very tired yet, he could not sleep at night nor rest in the day. His wife explained that she was at her wits end – she had tried everything. This gave the counsellor the opportunity to reframe the wife's shouting as a desperate attempt to help and to comment on the circular nature of their interactional sequence. The more he withdrew, the more she shouted, and the more he withdrew, the more she shouted and so on.

The counsellor focused on the fact that he had been very thrown by the information about his brother, and, in reply, the man volunteered that the thought was in his mind all the time. The counsellor suggested that the man's fury could be the disturbing thought. He reluctantly agreed with the counsellor that the information about his brother had made him so furious that he could not get it out of his mind, was easily distracted and could not concentrate or find any peace.

The counsellor explained that the patient had worked extremely hard to control all that was in his mind. He had busied himself, working harder and slowly exhausted himself. He had refused to talk about his feelings, but now, he was learning that his way of dealing with upset was not working. In the counselling sessions he was beginning to learn a new way. He spoke about the sense of injustice he felt about his brother not having the gene and the counsellor acknowledged that the fury was understandable. His inability to stop thinking about his disturbing feelings was likened to a record playing in his mind which was dominating his thoughts, pushing out everything else. However, the record was playing louder and he had lost control of it and could not switch off. He found this explanation entertaining as it was obviously a novel way of describing his experience. He and the counsellor began to establish a rather light-hearted attitude of acceptance of 'well we know how you do things, don't we?'

In the two further sessions the man learned to acknowledge his feelings and what emerged was his long-standing depression about his diagnosis (and fear of becoming like his father). Talking was extremely difficult for him, but he and the counsellor had found the almost humorous approach of 'Oh well, here we are again, doing what you hate, talking', suited him. He revealed that his dread of losing control and possibly becoming a burden to his family played on his mind. He confessed that he had decided that it would probably be better for his wife if they separated and further that once symptoms appeared, he felt he would end his life. Hearing this his wife became extremely angry and, through her tears, she angrily told him that she was his wife and under no circumstances was he to leave. He was touched by her anger but did not know how to respond. The counsellor, using the humorous approach they had developed said, 'I think she might care' and he cried.

He had been helped to see that he had spent a long time locking up his feelings about his own diagnosis. His anger had been building up, escalating and had become unmanageable after his brother's result. The counselling helped him discover his own feelings to find that underneath the disturbance lay fury and sadness. The man and wife left together – he reluctantly smiled and said he had found the discussions useful.

This is an example of how the problem seemed to start with the individual but the relationship between the couple had been simultaneously affected and had become the presenting difficulty. It is interesting that working with the relationship between the couple not only interrupted their pattern of escalating annoyance and withdrawal, but also helped undo a long-standing pattern of not expressing feelings. With a mixture of humour, interpretation and education, the counsellor had found a way of relating to the husband, helping with his expression of feelings and, as a result, facilitated an increased degree of intimacy and sharing between the couple.

This chapter has looked at the way the parts of a system interact and how the balance of the family system is destabilised by genetic knowledge which acts as another element needing to be included. The counsellor's entry into the family system forms the consultation system and helps the family understand their usual patterns and, in particular, how they have re-organised themselves around the potential for new information. The nature of the discussion helps them reflect and think about decision-making, change and processing emotions.

Systemic theory has been woven into the practice of genetic counselling with the counsellor thinking about the transgenerational pattern of relationships and, in particular, the dynamic around the genetic problem and the far reaching effect of genetic information. Understanding attachment patterns within a framework of systemic thought helps the counsellor in the various family groups. The examples present some important ways of working with families by observing and exploring who is present, how that decision was arrived at, how they interact together, the communication pattern and in particular how they deal with talking about painful issues. Exploring what happens *around* the genetic dilemma can free the family to think more constructively *about* the genetic dilemma.

Summary points

A family is a social system made up of individuals of different generations where the individuals are the inter-related parts, mutually affecting one another.

Genetic counselling and systemic thinking are intimately linked. The counsellor thinks systemically when exploring the systemic effect of the past and present relationships on the current dilemma. In addition, considering the effect of a test result on the immediate family is systemic thinking in the counsellor's everyday practice.

The family is always in the room, even if not actually present, alive within the individual as a physical and emotional memory influencing present thinking and behaviour.

A secure family is one which provides a reliable network of attachment relationships that enables the family members, of whatever age, to feel sufficiently secure to explore relationships with each other and with others outside the family. The motto of a secure family is 'collaborate to care'.

Information about a genetic disorder could be thought of as another element which needs to be included into the family system in the same way as a birth or death triggers an adjustment relating to the life cycle. Secure, flexible families can adapt to the information, whereas for insecurely attached families it can be the axis around which relationship difficulties or secrets arise.

Strategies which help support problem-solving include the resolution of conflict and support of the central couple relationship (Byng-Hall, 1995a). Working to resolve these issues creates the family's own secure base for thinking about genetic issues.

Working with parents and children

Awareness of the child in the consultation

This chapter continues with the theme of working with families, but in particular, the nuclear family and addresses the variety of ways parents and children come into genetic counselling. The counsellor will have gained an understanding of child development from clinical experience in paediatrics, general medicine or from the experience of being clinically involved with a number of children who have conditions which are genetically determined. It is not considered appropriate to give detailed theoretical points of child development from a cognitive or emotional perspective. Rather, the chapter begins with a general awareness of children as part of the consultation system before discussing how worries about children are considered in genetic counselling. Case examples will be presented which will demonstrate the salient points of family functioning around child problems and includes requests for testing children for adult-onset disorders.

When a child is the focus of a genetic consultation, he or she may be present in a consultation or, occasionally, parents may want to discuss their worries about their child in private. Alternatively there may be several children in a room as part of a consultation for a parent or a family. Young children can easily disrupt a consultation and some counsellors may prefer them to be looked after outside to ensure that the parents can concentrate and fully take part in the consultation. This may not be possible as a consultation is a potentially stressful encounter and children are often reluctant to leave a parent whom they sense is anxious.

The counsellor can prepare for a family who bring their children by having age-appropriate toys and drawing material available. This caters for young children and can help settle children and parents who do not want to be separated. As the consultation progresses and the tension drops, a child may feel free to wander away and play with another counsellor, either outside or inside the room but, equally, the way the children behave in the room can be informative.

The counsellor's awareness of the child begins with the initial greeting. Good practice begins with the counsellor making a personal introduction before looking to the adults to present themselves and finally making contact with the children. This introduction establishes the counsellor's respect for family hierarchy and endorses the parents as the carers of the children. The age of the children will determine the counsellor's behaviour. Very young children will want to stay close to a parent but, when the children are a little older, the counsellor may point out to the family group that there are toys and drawing material, making it clear that the child can use the play materials.

There are no fixed guidelines to help the counsellor work with different age groups and the chronological age may be deceptive, as emotional maturity and attachment dynamics play a part in how the child behaves. Whatever the age, the counsellor needs to have an awareness of everyone present in the consultation and begin by making explanatory statements. Children as young as 3-year-old are able to understand simple explanations and may settle more quickly if given an idea of what is happening. The counsellor can provide this and set the scene for the consultation with the following statement, 'I'm going to talk to your Mum and Dad for a while but we won't forget you and we'll stop at points to make sure you are all right'. With older children, it is important to ask or explain more about the focus of the interview, especially when the child is the focus of the consultation. Children as young as five or six can be asked, 'Did you know you were coming here today, or was it a surprise?' Or, 'Why do you think you Mum and Dad have brought you here today?' Further, if the child knows the reason for the referral, exploring how they were told and, by whom, gives valuable information about family culture and communication patterns. When the consultation concerns older children, it is important to actively involve them in the history and understanding of the disorder. If an interview concerns an older adolescent then the counsellor will need to treat them in an age-appropriate manner. For example, if a 15-year-old is the focus of the consultation, a counsellor can both recognise the adolescent's position and parental rights by a general comment such as, 'I believe we are going to talk about you today (speaking to young person). How should we begin? Would you like to start or shall I start with you (looking at the parents)?' With late teenagers, it may be important to ask if they want to be seen alone to respect their privacy. These different statements respect the child's development and cognitive ability.

Children may be content to play or draw and the counsellor may find that what they are drawing is related to the theme of the consultation or the mood of the family. Their behaviour has meaning, regardless of age. A child's behaviour is freer than an adult's and may give important clues about the atmosphere of the consultation and the family dynamics, especially attachment patterns. For example, a child's behaviour may be disruptive or the child may hover close to mother or father. Both can mean that they are aware of the tension in the room and are concerned about a parent or upset by the consultation. Even small babies react to atmosphere and pick up tension. An infant crying in a consultation may be responding to the build up of anxiety (which might have started before the beginning of a consultation). A child's crying is both a demand for attention and an indicator which can be a way of bringing care into the room. It is not always helpful to remove the crying child as seeing it as a signifier of distress is an opportunity to address the upset. In this way the counsellor is learning to read all behaviour as being an expression and a communication. When the adults in a family are becoming upset or tense, a simple statement to the children of, 'Mum and Dad are a bit worried about some things and they are trying to sort things out' is often useful. In addition, noticing a child come closer to a parent can be commented on with questions such as, 'Are you giving Mum a cuddle?' or 'Are you a bit worried about Mum?' That can then be followed by a simple explanation of the interview such as, 'We are talking about some worries to see if we can help'. The comments seem rather mundane and obvious but, to a child, it can make sense of confusion or fear and lets the child know that the counsellor is aware of everyone in the room. Alternatively, the counsellor may suggest to the parents that they explain what is being talked about. This encourages the adults to take responsibility for making sense of the world to children. In some families the parents naturally maintain their awareness of the children but, a consultation can also preoccupy parents such that they forget the children. Under such circumstances, the counsellor has to perform that role personally or, prompt the parents with helpful suggestions of explaining to the children, paying attention to their needs. The ability to talk directly to children in age appropriate terms, explaining their own dilemma or that of the family or individual adult, is an important attribute which a lot of parents have developed. However, if it is absent for whatever reason, the counsellor may have to take that role.

Every counsellor has been a child and will have personal experiences of childhood. These memories can colour and influence the counsellor's ability to talk to children of different ages. An interesting exercise for the counsellor is to explore what age child they find difficult to talk to and reflect on their own experience of that age. Memories might appear giving personal meaning or relevance to the difficulty.

The genetic disorder and parental overprotection

One of the developmental tasks for the family is to allow the child to move out of dependency to become an autonomous adult. The ability to launch the developing child into the world is a challenge for any family. The developmental path of the child involves negotiating several maturational hurdles: going to school, establishing peer contacts, working and creating another family. The detachment of the child from the parents is related to the parents' ability to let go and to say goodbye. As part of the growing-up process the parents have to tolerate the fact that their children may have different views. This is a mark of healthy development within the family. Families often get into difficulties around the challenge of the child becoming more separate and the difficulties can result in an interruption in the natural thrust of the child's maturational development and age-appropriate behaviour. The genetic counsellor will be interested in the influence of a genetic disorder on the family culture and child development. In particular, whether the gene has fostered a 'staying-close' family culture with children not separating (an enmeshed family), or alternatively, created a harsh 'distancing culture' with premature or inappropriate disengagement (a dismissive family). Neither enmeshment nor disengagement, the two poles of an insecure attachment pattern, facilitates the ability to think and feel, nor do they promote autonomy for the individual members.

When there is a genetic problem, the parents can understandably become overprotective and, in so doing, interrupt the developmental processes in a child. Families react differently to a child's disorder and some, because of anxiety, do not allow enough space for the child to be as normal as possible.

Rather, they foster a clinging relationship with the child. This is demonstrated in the following example.

Example

A mother requested an appointment in the genetic clinic as she was worried about her 7-year-old daughter. They had attended the genetic department on a number of occasions as the girl suffered from a skeletal dysplasia. She explained how frustrated she felt that her child cried so frequently and complained of being in such pain. She had to spend a considerable amount of time nursing her daughter and this cut across the time she had for her other children. She further described the helplessness she felt at not being able to put things right for her child and her despair that doctors could not diagnose the reason for the pain. She spoke about her tiredness, which at times she felt reached a point of total exhaustion and depression. She worked in the school her daughter attended – a job which was designed to stay close to her child to help her. The counsellor wondered about this idea and asked the mother if she thought staying close to the child all the time was useful. This was followed by an invitation for the mother to think about what going to school meant. There was agreement that school was not just for education, as it had the additional function of helping the child mature. That meant letting the child find some way of coping with being alone and growing-up. The separation needed for the child to go to school has the function of encouraging the child to manage without mother's constant presence and subsequently triggers further emotional development. The woman found this conversation useful and explained that she needed to hear that she was not being neglectful to let go her child a little. She was invited to reflect on the nature of her relationship with all her children and whether having a child with difficulties had affected her relationship with that particular child. She freely acknowledged how she overprotected the child with the disorder and was self-critical of this tendency, knowing somehow that it might not be helping. She felt she had to compensate in some way as she found her child's disorder extremely difficult to accept. She spoke of feeling extremely sad at her child's dilemma, guilty that, in her eyes, she had given her child such a difficult life, yet annoyed with her child for being so demanding. At times in the consultation she laughed at herself and, at other times, she was tearful. The counsellor commented that the mother and her daughter were both in pain.

The counsellor reminded the woman that she had begun the consultation with her concerns that her child complained of pain and asked what ideas she might have. The woman volunteered that the child certainly had difficulties but, she wondered whether there was something else going on between them and asked, 'Is she playing me up because I'm too soft on her?' The counsellor replied by suggesting that it seemed that she had been asking herself that question for some time.

With further enquiry about the family, the counsellor learned that the woman's husband frequently told her to stop fussing over the child. When asked whether she agreed with her husband that she did fuss the child, she laughingly answered she did, but she did not listen. The counsellor's response was also to laugh and to say that her laughter gave the game away and maybe she and her husband could think about their management of their child together.

Clearly the problem presented begs the question of where the boundary of a genetic consultation lies. The problem is not directly genetic but the woman had a high regard for the genetic counsellor and understandably brought her anxiety and frustration to the genetic clinic. The interview demonstrated that having a psychological understanding of attachment patterns and child development can enable a counsellor to be effective in helping and alleviating distress in one thoughtful interview. The interview content is interesting as the counsellor does not address the symptom of the child's distress directly, but focuses the discussion on the relationships around the problem and how the mother and child had become so closely paired together. The counsellor's light closing intervention attempted to redress the family relationships by placing the couple relationship as the main pairing. The latter is an example of undoing triangulation in a family to re-establish the appropriate pairing. When a child is overprotected, not only is that child's development interrupted but, in addition, the family relationships also become unbalanced. There is an overemphasis on the parent/child relationship and a marginalising of the couple relationship. Detaching the mother from her over-involvement with the child, frees her to be involved with her husband. Looking at it another way, the child is freed to develop if the mother attaches to her husband.

A family who have a child with any disorder is challenged to adjust and cope and, as described in Chapter 2, that involves acknowledging and processing the disappointment, grief and other emotions which may arise. Processing these emotions to achieve a balance of acceptance to live within the limitations of the disorder is an enormous task for parents, the affected child and other siblings. The mother in this example was able to express her annoyance and frustration. In accepting these feelings, the counsellor prevented the mother from acting-out the feelings by rejecting the child or, the opposite, overprotecting. The parental adjustment and processing of mixed emotions is an important element in the child's personal adjustment.

A child's self-image is an internal concept built-up over time and begins in the mirror of the mother's eyes where the image the child receives is a reflection of the mother's thoughts. It is not difficult for a child to pick-up anxiety or lack of acceptance. The child continues to need varying degrees of environmental support to achieve a mastery of the maturational hurdles of development and increase self-confidence.

In a single consultation the counsellor established a particular kind of conversation which enabled the mother to review her relationship with her child and speculate about its unhelpful aspects. The concepts in the counsellor's mind were not diagnostic trying to make sense of the child's pain and, very interestingly, neither did the mother seem to want a diagnosis. The mother was as concerned as the counsellor about her relationship with her child. It would be presumptuous to predict a change in the child's experience of pain. The obvious result of the interview was that it validated the idea of mother letting her child have more space, in the hope that the child would mature and learn, as far as possible, to manage some of her difficulties.

The interview did not give the mother any new information, but it allowed her to think about what she already knew. This is an example of how the genetic counsellor can make constructive interventions based on an understanding of how the family's attachment/detachment dynamic needs to change in relationship to the developmental needs of the child members. These psychological interventions can prevent the genetic disorder interrupting the child's developmental process and alleviate distress in parents.

Blaming a child's emotional problem on the genetic disorder

The counsellor is sometimes drawn into a family dilemma about a child, particularly when the genetic problem is blamed for the child's difficulty. The disorder can be a convenient peg to hang a problem but, although this is understandable, such a strategy can block the family's problem-solving ability. With an understanding of family functioning, the counsellor is equipped to assess the factors involved in the problem and the contribution of the genetic condition.

Example

A family asked for a consultation as they were very worried about their 15-year-old son who was refusing to go to school. They were well-known to the genetic department as of their son had a genetically determined disorder which needed monitoring. One of the characteristics of the disorder resulted in the boy looking unusual. As in the last example, this raises the appropriateness of the genetic department being involved in a problem of school refusal. However, a genetic counsellor is frequently a trusted emotional resource for families and, with specialist knowledge of a disorder, may be able to help a young person who is struggling with looking different. Adolescence is a challenging time for the whole family. The young person is struggling with issues relating to identity and autonomy and can be very lonely. It is important for the young person who is detaching from the family to have a sense of belonging to a peer group and looking different can result in exclusion.

The counsellor began by acknowledging that the family had made contact as they had some concerns and asked, 'How might I be able to help you?' 'Who would like to start?' The mother stated the problem of her son's non-attendance at school and was forcefully interrupted by her son who said, 'I'm not going'. The mother continued with her story of her son complaining that he had been bullied at school, as he looked a bit different. The boy angrily stated 'That's nothing to do with it, everyone gets bullied, I hate school'. The boy explained he was not worried about looking different and wanted to go out to work. That led to a discussion about how both parents worked very hard in their jobs but wanted something better for their children. They regretted they had not done well in school and, to their dismay; none of their three children did any work in school. The counsellor asked if the parents had to chase the children to do their work and received a surprising answer from the father. He started to laugh and explained that the children were never chased to do anything. Rather, they had their own way all of the time, were never asked to help in the house, had no responsibilities and he and his wife did everything for them. In addition, they never left the children alone in the house. It emerged that there were no routines of bedtime for the younger children or responsibilities for the older boy. With amusement the father said that he thought that in their family there were no rules, the children were in charge and they, the parents, were slaves. 'It's funny really as my wife was the class bully and she still bullies me, but she spoils the children.' This comment resulted in the mother also laughing. The counsellor put a positive construction on 'the slavery' by saying that the couple obviously cared about their children, but it raised the question of how to help children mature and whether bullying, or spoiling, was helpful. The mother answered by saying, 'I don't know what to do, he has everything he wants, I do everything for him and his brothers'. The consultation continued with the couple discussing how they felt they were faced with a dilemma they could not solve and that it might be related to the fact that they as parents had no power to help or control their children. The counsellor reframed their depression and their son's behaviour and said, 'I know this all seems rather hopeless to you at the moment but I wonder whether your son is in some way doing you all a favour. His challenge is inviting you to really think very hard about limits and organisation in your family and, in some way, is making sure that you two, as parents, work together to address these issues'. That comment seemed to support the parental couple and the conversation moved to them exploring how they might begin to do things differently and what might help. Although the parents had found the consultation helpful, there was a conclusion that the family would benefit from ongoing specialist help.

This consultation was extremely worrying as clearly the family had serious difficulties in their general family functioning. The genetic problem did not appear to have contributed to the family's difficulties. As a result of the consultation, the school refusal was not seen as connected to the genetic difficulty, but was considered to be in the context of the family structural problems of no hierarchy, boundaries or separateness. The family was working hard to provide and offer the best they could for their children, but they had lost their authority and structure and were confused about how to help their children.

Unravelling family conflict around testing for a genetic disorder

The genetic counsellor frequently witnesses family conflict in consultations. In the following example the conflict is around testing teenage boys for a familial cancer which had appeared at an early age in several members of the father's family. The parents asked for a consultation in the hope that the counsellor would be able to persuade both boys of the wisdom of being tested. This would suggest to a counsellor that there was some family conflict around the boys being tested. However, initially it would be important to understand the disorder, the family's factual knowledge and how the children had been told. The nature of the disorder would give the counsellor an understanding of the request and whether the parental idea of testing the boys was based on anxiety or more medically determined.

The consultation began with introductions and the history of the disorder. The mother was the main spokesperson, with the father agreeing and seeming actively-involved. The counsellor then spoke to Andrew the older boy and asked when he had been told about the family history. The conversation continued as follows.

Andrew: Last week.

Counsellor: I'd like to hear a bit about that and how it was for you.
Andrew: Mum said you've got to be tested. She got all bossy, telling me what to do, as usual.

Counsellor: Was that the first time you were told about the problem in your father's family?

Andrew: No, we all knew that some of Dad's family had been operated on and that Dad went for check-ups.

Counsellor: So you sort of knew but didn't.

Andrew: Yes, but we never talk about it.

Counsellor: Tell me a bit more about last week.

Andrew: Well they decided to talk about it, for a change, and said 'you've got to be tested'. I just said 'No', I'm fed up of being told what to do all the time.

Counsellor: What happened after that?

Andrew: My mother started shouting and I shouted back.

Counsellor: And was your father there?

Andrew: Yes.

Counsellor (turning to the father): When your wife and son started to argue what did you do?

Father: I tried to settle them down.

Counsellor: And did you succeed?

Father: Not really, Andrew stormed out of the room and my wife started to cry.

Counsellor (speaking to Peter the second son): Were you part of this discussion or were you told at another time?

Peter: Yes, I was there and Dad explained that it was a way of making sure I'm looked after properly.

Counsellor (speaking to mother): Is that how you thought it happened?

Mother: No, not really, I can't say anything to Andrew without him getting angry.

Counsellor: So let me see if I understand this correctly. You boys were told together and Mum and Andrew had a row which Dad tried to settle down, but Andrew left. What I don't know is whether Peter was told it would help to be tested before Andrew left or after?

Father: After.

Counsellor to Andrew: Did you know why your mother wanted you to be tested?

Andrew: Of course I did, I'm not stupid.

Counsellor: Do you have more rows with Mum and Dad than Peter?

Andrew: Yes, they go on at me all the time. They don't treat me like a 17-year-old. They just don't trust me.

Counsellor (to both parents): What's your view about that?

Mother: I'm only trying to help him but he's so independent, you can't tell him anything.

Counsellor: Let me have another go at understanding this. Mum thinks Andrew is independent and Andrew wants to be independent. So when Mum tries to help Andrew thinks she is going on at him. Father tries to help but Andrew leaves and Peter has the explanation of the family trying to care for the boys correctly. Quite a struggle isn't it and Andrew ends up thinking you don't trust him.
Father: I hope the boy will see sense and not just argue for the sake of it.

Counsellor: What do you think Andrew?
Andrew: If they would leave me alone and stop treating me like a child, of course I'll have the test, I'm not stupid, they just think I am.

This extract demonstrates the counsellor tracking the interaction and gently teasing out the meaning of everyone's behaviour, listening to everyone's story and putting it together, highlighting the whole interactional sequence. The counsellor's task was not to persuade both boys to be tested, but to clarify the family dynamics.

Difficulty telling the children

In the following example the counsellor is asked to see a couple who were depressed and had difficulty speaking to each other and to their children about the husband's family history.

Example

A couple had recently moved to the area and were referred to the genetic department as the father had polycystic kidney disease. He had recently had a kidney transplant operation and the surgical team were concerned about the couple and the family as a whole. They all seemed depressed and unable to talk about the genetic nature of the disorder. The counsellor made contact in the immediate post-operative period and followed up with an outpatient appointment sometime later. In the beginning of that consultation the counsellor established the family history and learnt that of the husband's long-standing and frequent illness prior to his transplant. The couple presented as people who had difficulty sharing their feelings together; the wife was upset and the husband withdrawn, leaving a huge space between them. Rather than make the observation, the counsellor asked if they had different ways of coping with the strain and worry of the husband's illness. The wife eagerly described their difference and the counsellor then asked how were they able to support and comfort one another. The question was met with the wife glancing at the husband, but no reply was forth coming. The counsellor asked how much it had affected them as a family and was told that they never spoke about their situation. The wife explained that they did not talk much and that was how it was.

The counsellor tried to engage the husband but he dismissed the significance of speaking by saying, 'What's the point, there's nothing to be done? I've had a transplant, leave it at that, it's all over'. The counsellor wondered if it was all over and asked what they both needed now and what the children knew. The wife became very upset and explained some of the long-standing worries around her husband's illness. She could not think of telling the children, as that would be too painful; she did not want to hurt them. The counsellor wondered whether she was speaking about her own pain or the children's and continued by asking which would harm them the most, 'knowing', or 'not knowing'. The wife understood that she was protecting the children, but the husband remained silent. The exploration moved to what the children had been told when their father had been hospital. The wife revealed that no explanation had been given. She agreed that the children were possibly a bit worried, but she wanted to keep the family as normal as possible. The counsellor understood the natural desire to protect children from any worries and that breaking bad news sometimes felt like shattering a child's innocence. The counsellor continued by making the educative comment that even very young children know when something is wrong and, that it was easier for children to have a worry spoken about than kept a secret. It was explained that silence could be frightening. When there are no explanations, thoughts and worries, coloured by imagination, can go around in a child's head in a confused way. The wife seemed to be supported by this educative approach.

The consultation then moved to exploring how the father had been told about his family history and he replied that he was told after his mother's death. Rather pointedly he was asked whether looking back he might have preferred to have known sooner. He replied that it might have saved a lot of trouble. The counsellor left the couple to think about how becoming aware of that thought would alter his decision of when he passed on the information to his children.

This interview explored the family culture of dealing with worries and used an educative approach to explain that children already know when something worrying is going on. Further, it helps to have an adult clarify the reality. It also explored the dynamic between the couple and the intergenerational communication pattern of giving genetic information. This resulted in the husband acknowledging that he would have liked to have known his family history earlier.

The counsellor's entry into the family system supported and understood the couple's dilemma so providing a secure-enough place for exploration. The counsellor did not find it easy to relate to the father, but direct questioning around his experiences produced valuable information.

The testing of children for adult-onset disorders

The genetic testing of a symptomatic child to confirm a medical diagnosis or testing to establish the presence of a disorder where the child would benefit from ongoing medical care does not pose an ethical problem. Equally, if an under-age adolescent has instigated the request and is deemed sufficiently mature, again there is no problem, although the assessment of maturity is complex (Binedell et al., 1996; Sarangi and Clarke, 2002). However, the predictive testing of children for adult-onset disorders, where the child does not stand to benefit and is too young to participate in decision-making is more problematic. Balancing a parent's right to know against respecting the autonomy and privacy rights of the child can be very complex. The parental argument would be that knowledge would remove any uncertainty about the disorder being present or absent. They would be able to decide when to give the information and consequently, facilitate a better psychosocial adjustment. That point of view can be countered by the need to protect the child's privacy and autonomy and testing could impact on child's upbringing in a negative way.

The testing of children has been a topic of debate for some time (Clarke and Flinter, 1996; Michie, 1996) and has led to the production of Guidelines for genetic testing of healthy children by the Canadian Paediatric Society (2003). With the best interests of the child in mind, testing of healthy children for adult-onset disorders, where there is no benefit to the child, is controversial. Similarly, testing to determine the carrier status of a child where it would be of purely reproductive significance is not recommended.

Within this framework, there is still different individual practice and there will be healthy children tested. There would appear to be agreement that a blanket refusal is unhelpful and it could lead to a reactive determination by some parents. Each request for testing of a child needs to be taken individually and the debate put in a balanced manner. This involves a counsellor listening to the parents' request and understanding their thinking, whilst balancing it with the ethical dilemma of the child's autonomy and rights. This thoughtful counselling and open debate may in itself be beneficial to families. It provides an opportunity for the parents to think about the meaning of the disorder and the implications of this arising in their child.

The following examples do not attempt to enter the debate of the wisdom of testing or not testing. They illustrate counselling experiences which demonstrate different presentations of this dilemma and the counselling strategies which are used to facilitate thinking and debate.

Examples

A father's attempt to protect his child from experiencing a disappointment similar to his own

A couple, where the father has polycystic kidney disease, brought their young baby to the genetic department. The father told the counsellor that the infant was healthy and 'she's been scanned and it didn't show anything …' He continued, 'I was wondering whether or not she could be tested now and if you could tell me, one way or another, whether or not she has polycystic kidneys?' The counsellor explored the family context of the request and was told by the father that as a young man he had failed a medical examination for entry to the police force on the grounds of his kidney problem. 'I knew nothing about it until then. I tried to find my father, he left my mother when I was a baby and I learnt that he had died of kidney disease. So it was a complete shock to me.' He movingly described his disappointment by saying '… it broke my heart at 18'.

The counsellor and the father continued to discuss the pros and cons of testing the baby. The counsellor explained how the child's health could be monitored by blood pressure and kidney function observations. The father responded and explained 'That's the difficulty … worrying unnecessary, every year for the next 16 years … I don't want to be coming to the hospital all the time'. He continued, 'if it was necessary, she'd be here … But for me, without knowing one way or another, it's too much; it's something I don't want in my family life unless she has a problem. … Every year coming here … it's something we want to go away'. He clarified that 'it's so we can prepare ourselves … and that I'd like to have it straight in my mind'. 'I don't want to accept it for her.' In a moment of deep reflection he said '… It's difficult and maybe I'm not taking all her interests at heart, but I want to know one way or another'.

The theme of a broken heart was mentioned several times; sometimes the father referred to his own heart, at others he spoke of his wife's heart but he stressed '… I wouldn't want **her** heart being broken', referring to his daughter.

These extracts of the conversation between the counsellor and the family reveal the amount of anguish the father felt. Hospital visits for monitoring would be a reminder that his child could have the same disorder as himself and that she may have to confront the same issues. The over-riding theme was that the father did not want his daughter to have her heart broken and prevented from fulfilling a dream. His greatest desire was to protect his child from future emotional pain and to relieve himself and his wife from the pain of uncertainty.

The counsellor had a considerable task of laying the debate in front of the family and working within the context of the particular experiences and individual life story. The most obvious intervention for the genetic counsellor was educative, presenting the ethical dilemma of balancing the child's right to privacy against the parents' right to know and, to observe the effect of that educative intervention. The theme which repeatedly emerged in the consultation was the man's personal disappointment of his dream being frustrated and his desire to protect his child from a similar grief. This led the counsellor to concentrate on a more psychological approach and to make an empathic statement such as 'You are telling me something about your own emotional pain and your desire to protect your child from a similar experience'. The man continued to talk about his disappointment and the effect it had on his life. He thought he had got over it but his upset had been resurrected by his child's vulnerability. It would be important to know how the man coped with disappointment in general and, in particular, how he would cope with the disappointment if his child tested positive. Such a conversation would be exploring a past grief and preparing for a possible future grief. His statement of 'I don't want to accept it for her' suggests he is almost refusing to acknowledge it as a possibility. The counsellor might want to understand more about what he meant by his expression of repeated hospital visits being 'too much'. It suggests a concern about being able to cope. Talking about the fear is a way of entering it and the genetic counsellor is an ideal companion to help accompany him.

The simplest response to the father's request would be for the counsellor to agree to the child being tested as it is only human to want to relieve the man of such intense pain. However his desperation for a negative result suggests he is unprepared for the reverse. The risk in testing is that the father could become more disturbed. It would seem advisable to help him grieve for his own disappointment, before making any further decision.

Invoking the voice of the child

This example is of a couple who have lost several pregnancies as a result of early miscarriages. The cause had been linked to the presence of a balanced chromosome rearrangement in the father leading to an unbalanced chromosome complements in some sperm, rendering the conceptions non-viable. The couple have two children; a son, who had not been tested and a younger daughter, who had been tested in foetal life and found to be clear of both the balanced and unbalanced rearrangement. The father was now seeking testing of the 6-year-old son to clarify whether he was a carrier.

In the consultation the counsellor explained the complexity of the situation and the need to consider the rights of the child, especially as it referred to the child's future reproductive life. The counsellor asked the father to reflect and consider 'How would you raise it with him?' The response from the father was that he had various plans of how to take blood for another reason and concluded, 'I think that the only way is to cover it up with a 6-year-old'. It transpired that the family had tried on a number of occasions to persuade doctors to take blood for the genetic assessment when the child had been ill and so far had failed.

The counsellor continued inviting the couple to imagine the scene, 'and when it came back, what would you do with the result?' The reply was 'If it came back as a problem we would leave it initially, because of his age … we would leave it until he was 16, or when he starts courting, when he's old enough to really understand'. The father explained his thinking behind the request by explaining 'It might be easier to test at this age now, when we can say you have to have the blood test done. Whereas if we left testing till he is 14 or older, he might start saying "No" and that's the end of the story'. The counsellor again attempted to help the father consider the consequences and asked, 'How would you tell him and how might he react?' 'You know your son … but I have some reservations about doing something too surreptitiously. How do you think he would take it?' The father justified keeping the information from the boy by arguing that he was very intelligent and sensitive and would worry about it.

This is an extremely challenging interview where the counsellor used the technique of taking up 'the voice of the child', whose opinion is not being considered. The father had a number of rationalisations and arguments to justify his thinking. The counsellor introduced imaginary scenarios, projecting the father into the future, dramatising the family scene to include the boy's voice and generally heightening the importance of the decision. The counsellor subsequently relinquished that unilateral position and handed the idea of his son back to the father, by saying again 'You know your son …' In so doing the polarity in the session then changed. Having invited the father to imagine the son's reaction to testing, the counsellor then retreated and left the dilemma with the parent.

The art of using the technique of introducing an unheard voice lies in the ability of the counsellor to let go at some point. Continuing to hold the position of the absent voice would have been oppositional and argumentative. It would have resulted in the counsellor falling into the trap of acting-out a child/parent conflict.

Other interventions could include exploring the parents' difficulty in waiting when it was not an immediate health issue or reframing the father's request as a way of trying to protect and do the best for his son. The latter would pave the way to allow the counsellor to hold both the rights of the son and the father in mind. For example, the counsellor might say, 'On the one hand, I understand your concern and your anxiety to look after your son; on the other hand, I am also trying to imagine your son's viewpoint'. If the counsellor can hold both ideas in mind, then this introduces the possibility of the balance being found in the father.

A child of a separated couple and is he like his father

A mother, who had left her son's father, wanted to know whether the boy had inherited his father's genetic potential for a muscle disorder, so raising the general issue of whether the son was like his father. Life with the boy's father had been acrimonious and, after many years of a difficult relationship, the couple had separated very traumatically. The woman was still carrying very negative feelings about the boy's father. She was understandably worried that her son might have to suffer in the future if he had his father's disorder.

The mother was counselled and given the reasoning for not testing her son at his young age. This seemed to settle her and she went away, only to return a year later for the counsellor to go through the debate again. This happened on three separate occasions and each time she went away, seemingly satisfied with the conclusion of not testing. However, on the fourth occasion, the counsellor did not put forward the balanced view of reasoning around testing children for adult-onset disorders. The counsellor agreed to test the child and the mother rejected the offer.

How can this change of heart are understood? One hypothesis would be that the mother had concerns about her son's future as a constant background worry which she needed to talk about, hence the repeated visits. Another hypothesis would be that the mother was ambivalent, wanting and not wanting to know. By consulting with a counsellor that internal debate becomes externalised and becomes two different voices. However, as soon as the counsellor changes and no longer takes up the balancing position but agrees with her, the woman has to consider the whole dilemma within herself.

It is interesting to think about the repetitive nature of the interaction with the woman requesting and the counsellor refusing. That interaction would then trigger more of the same, persistence and resistance. However, once the resistance is removed, the woman has to reconsider her position. This is a well-established technique of the counsellor not continuing to counter the individual's argument. Indeed, holding a very firm position can be counter-productive and result in increasing the force of the demand. In the example presented the timing of the removal of the resistance to testing was obviously a masterful stroke of experience, knowing that to continue would produce more of the same dynamic.

These requests for the testing of children are a particular challenge to the counsellor who has the dilemma of juggling the wisdom of experience, a non-directive stance and holding in mind the debate about the rights of parents and those of the child.

Summary points

The counsellor can prepare for a family and children by having age-appropriate toys and drawing material available. The counsellor's awareness of the child begins with the initial greeting. Good practice begins with the counsellor making a personal introduction and then looking for the adults to present themselves, before making contact with the children. This introduction establishes the counsellor's respect for family hierarchy of the parents as the carers of the children.

A counsellor's approach needs to respect the child's development, cognitive ability and to provide age appropriate explanations.

All behaviour has meaning; it is an expression and a communication. An infant crying in a consultation is a demand for attention and can be a way of bringing care into the room.

Good counselling techniques and an understanding of families and children enable a counsellor to therapeutically intervene in one interview to help families disentangle relationship problems from genetic related problems.

8

The influence of the nature of the disorder on the consultation

The previous chapters have focused on different aspects of the genetic counselling encounter and have put particular emphasis on the importance of the uniqueness of the individual or family. The counsellor respects that uniqueness by offering an appropriately attuned and facilitating relationship which forms the solid core of a consultation. It determines how the consultation proceeds and is the context within which the different genetic consultations take place. There may be a single consultation where the emphasis changes at different stages of the counselling process, or several meetings with a different emphasis in each one. This chapter begins with a common framework which can be applied to all genetic counselling. It moves to focusing on how four different disorders, by their very nature and their implications, will influence the focus and process of the interview and, consequently, the emphasis placed by the counsellor.

The common denominators which apply to all consultations

Genetic counselling may appear to revolve around a central element of information both giving and receiving, but the process does not follow a straight line of an individual asking a question which is then answered. The counsellor makes a series of interventions and the way the individual or family responds will determine the subsequent direction. The counsellor is constantly observing responses and reviewing and adjusting the path of the consultation correspondingly. For instance, the process begins with a question being asked and that may take the form of a symptom, a worry, a request for information or many other forms. If this is likened to the patient bringing a parcel into the consultation arena, then the first intervention is an exploration of that parcel to discover what is inside. The counsellor observes the responses to the exploration. At some point the counsellor will make another intervention which may clarify the family history, analyse ways of dealing with stress and identify characteristic coping and attachment patterns. The counsellor observes what happens as this story unfolds and may have to respond to emerging problems, which may result in the genetic counselling process taking a different path. The counsellor makes a further intervention by giving general information about genetic inheritance and particular information about the disorder under discussion. This is the beginning of discussing individual risk and again the process may be diverted or halted by the response to the intervention. In summary, the pattern of the overall process of genetic counselling is not a straight line. It is a series of spirals, where each circle is observing and auditing the last intervention. The result of this constant auditing means that the formulation of the meaning of the original question may be quite different from its initial appearance and, as a result, the consultation may take a winding path to its conclusion.

Consultations in different disorders

Within this general framework, the nature of the different disorders will influence the consultation not only in content, but also because each disorder has different implications and consequences, with different options open to the individual. The counsellor's sensitivity to the implication of each disorder determines how a consultation is focused and where there is a need for particular delicacy. This chapter demonstrates similarities and differences in genetic clinics which specialise in four different areas: prenatal, cancer, Huntington's disease and dysmorphology and discusses how the counsellor adjusts the consultations correspondingly.

The nature of the disorder, the number of consultations and the time element

The prenatal and dysmorphology clinics have any number of disorders to consider and, most often, the discussions are about what has already happened, with the uncertainty focused on the implications of the disorder. In prenatal clinics, there may be a number of consultations and these can have a sense of urgency as there is the possibility of terminating a pregnancy and the need to make a decision within a time limit. In both cancer and Huntington's disease there is one condition to consider although the site of the cancer may vary. Transmission is by an autosomal-dominant gene with complete penetrance in the latter and testing is most likely to be presymptomatic. In Huntington's disease the initial uncertainty is about presence of the gene and, in those who have tested positive, uncertainty changes to *when* and not *if* the disease will appear. In contrast, in cancer genetics, a positive test result still carries varying degrees of uncertainty as other factors come into play. The implications of having information in these two conditions have resulted in a number of consultations being recommended. These have been put together as a protocol. The time interval built into the protocol allows for the digestion and emotional processing of the information before the formulation of a decision to be tested.

The implications of the disorders

All of these conditions have serious implications for the families and, understandably, the consultations are emotionally highly charged. In the prenatal clinics, the most upsetting area centres on the possibility of a child having an abnormality and, sometimes, that raises the extremely difficult decision of possible termination of the pregnancy.

Cancer carries enormous fear of pain and death which is sometimes based on fact, but may include projected fears and fantasies. Huntington's disease is a late-onset disorder which is debilitating and disabling with a florid presentation of changes in mental state and behaviour. In dysmorphology the distress of the disorder relates to the difference from the average person and the fact that it is visible. In addition, there may be implications related to the associated elements of a syndrome and these may necessitate treatment or educational help. However, the main challenges are psychological and involve attitude, acceptance, self-image and identity.

The possibility of treatment for the disorder

An important factor in an individual's reactions to having personal genetic knowledge is related to the possibility of treatment of the disorder. In the prenatal clinics, the importance of the diagnosis and implications for the future life of the foetus will be an important factor in determining the future of the pregnancy. There is an important difference between the presymptomatic diagnosis of Huntington's disease and cancer. To date, in the former the development of the condition cannot be averted; but in the latter, prognosis can be significantly influenced by monitoring which offers early detection of cancer. This difference probably explains the different uptake figures for testing of 10% for Huntington's disease, 50% for breast cancer and 80% for familial adenomatous polyposis (Meiser et al., 2000). In dysmorphology, plastic surgery may be used to correct the disfigurement, but treatment is mainly related to the associated disorders.

The status of the couple

In all four disorders there will be an effect beyond the affected individual as very often a partner or spouse is involved in the consultation process. Indeed, in predictive testing it is considered helpful for a close relative to be present for support, especially for a test result. Partners will be affected personally by a test result and their attitude may influence a decision to be tested. Kessler (1993), in his article 'Forgotten Person in the Huntington Disease Family' has written about the impact of the diagnosis of Huntington's disease on the 'important other', highlighting the many different responses evoked in the partner. The status of the couple is different in the prenatal dilemma as theoretically there is joint ownership of the foetus. Similarly, as dysmorphology usually is concerned with a child, the status of the couple is different and both parents may be involved in the consultation.

The counsellor's emphasis

From these similarities and differences in the four specialist areas of genetic counselling, it can be seen that although information-giving is common to all, the implications for each disorder will necessitate the counsellor emphasising different aspects. In Huntington's disease clinics, the aim will be to facilitate a full exploration of the implications of having a result; in the cancer genetic clinic the goal is likely to be directed towards high uptake; in the prenatal clinic one of the main goals will be to inform and to facilitate decision-making by working with the couple as a unit; in dysmorphology the initial focus will be on making an accurate diagnosis and identifying any associated aspects which need attention. In addition, each condition produces particular psychological challenges which will also direct the counsellor's behaviour. These differences will be considered separately.

Considering the details of the four specialities

Prenatal clinic

Women who attend for prenatal genetic counselling fall into four main groups: those who have had a previous handicapped child; those who do not have a handicapped child but a positive family history of genetic disorder; older women (over 35); and those who have had a positive screening test (Green and Statham, 1996). In theory, women from the first two groups will have prior knowledge, be less shocked and have done some mental rehearsal and emotional preparation. In contrast, when the abnormality is picked-up as a result of screening, there will have been no emotional preparation and the situation may be a complete shock. In their analysis Evers-Kiebooms et al. (1988) found that women having a test on the grounds of age are less anxious than those in the other groups. Women are not always clear about screening and therefore are ill-prepared for a result. A number of workers have emphasised the importance of misinformation or inadequate information and have reported that it appeared to increase worry and anxiety. When there is the possibility of further diagnostic testing, there is often a tension between wanting the certainty of a diagnosis, but there is a fear of an invasive test and the possibility of a test induced miscarriage (Kenen et al., 2000). The distress of the situation is compounded by a sense of urgency if a termination is being considered and this can affect not only the patients, but also the counsellors and the quality of the consultation.

In prenatal clinics, educative genetic counselling, prior to a diagnostic procedure, will be directed towards clarifying what is already known, what is unclear, what would change with a diagnostic intervention and if the procedure could affect the pregnancy. At this stage the psychological intervention will be directed towards containing anxiety so that information can be absorbed and a decision made. After the diagnostic procedure, the thrust of the educative intervention will be to provide information about the nature of the abnormalities and the effect they will have on the future life of the unborn child. The psychological interventions will be directed towards facilitating the emotional processing in the parents who will be coping with a result and its implications. There may be a need for further discussions if the future of the pregnancy is in doubt.

The degree of emotional pain and the added intensity in these clinics are linked to the fact that a future child is involved. Symbolically, the foetus is an everyday miracle of life created by individuals, representing their love. Abnormalities in this area can be regarded as an attack on the individual's creativity and an interruption of the sense of immortality carried in the future generations. The fact that a child is involved easily engages a counsellor's compassion and empathy. This is essential for the success of the consultation, but in this area there is possibly a greater risk that the counsellor will be over-involved or identify with the grieving parents.

The counsellor uses many different educational strategies to make sure that the information is scientific and objective. Facts and figures are presented simply, the counsellor frequently talking in general terms about 'babies with this problem' rather than 'your baby'. This strategy depersonalises the situation and has the potential to defuse high emotionality. It also invites a more reflective stance. This educative intervention is not a one-off statement as it may need to be repeated and explained in different ways to address any areas of confusion and misperception. The counsellor and patients have different approaches to the information; whereas the counsellor attempts to remain scientific and logical in presenting information; the patients concerned are more likely to be geared towards the reduction of uncertainty at a psychological level (Sarangi et al., 2003). The counsellor's logical and factually based responses are constantly trying to balance and correct distortions which are generated by the patient's psychological misperceptions. The cognitive misinterpretation will be related to the patient's emotional style and results in the counsellor balancing a minimising style of disregarding the significance of the information by emphasising and heightening the intensity. In contrast, where the significance is being exaggerated emotionally or factually, the counsellor will be balancing with more levelling statements. These educative interventions are factual, but they are also designed to affect psychological changes in perception.

In addition, the counsellor will need interventions and skills which are more purely psychologically based. Lippman (1999) explored how women discussed pregnancy, age, Down's syndrome and prenatal testing in the context of their responses to offers of amniocentesis. The exploration revealed how the information became woven into experiences and understandings of feelings and beliefs and became 'embodied knowledge', which the woman owned. The implications are for the counsellor to refine listening skills and to be alert to the individual's use of information in the context of their life experiences. The recommendation is for a rapprochement of educational and psychological approaches rather than providing more and more information.

In this highly emotional area the counsellor needs to be able to tolerate the degree of distress without becoming professionally mechanistic, overwhelmed, over-involved or too helpful. Working through the upset with a couple is complicated as each individual has to personally process the emotions and consider the feelings of the other partner. An abnormal foetus challenges the internal resources of both individuals involved and the experience of shock, grief, anxiety and disappointment can seriously affect the relationship between the couple. The degree of intimacy may enable them to be close to one another, to share and understand each other's hurt and to communicate that either through words, gesture or touch. This is the mark of a sophisticated, mature, relationship of concern and regard for the self and for the other. However, intimacy and the ability to understand 'the other' are sometimes outside an individual's repertoire. Even if intimacy is normally present, it can be compromised when the challenge of the situation exposes the relationship to intense stress. Alternatively, the crisis may be an opportunity. The distress can break down long-established barriers and enable defences to open up, facilitating a new closer relationship. This can happen when a couple, who are normally reserved, find their grief unites them.

If a couple has, or can find, this ability to be close, then this exchange of pain and understanding can comfort and support both individuals and may ease their distress. In addition, if there is an issue about the future of the pregnancy, the couple will find it easier to make a decision if the bond between them is strong and also if they have a sense of joint ownership and acceptance.

Most of the time couples or individuals find their way through the difficulties which confront them; they carry their disappointments in the way they know best. However, the genetic counsellor is a key factor in facilitating an interview where the couple are experiencing some difficulty between them.

The genetic counsellor's role is to provide a secure-enough base and a framework for the couple to work through their emotions. In earlier chapters it has been clarified that the key element in the counsellor's ability to provide a secure-enough base is the ability to understand and to empathise with the patient's subjective experience. When the counsellor is working with a couple, the task of empathising is with both partners, each viewpoint, including the difficulty they have in their relationship. This even-handed approach can at times be difficult, especially where the difference between the couple is such that it is easier to personally identify with one member and not the other. Under that circumstance the therapeutic potential in remaining neutral is lost. In particular, it may be easier for the counsellor to understand the perspective of the partner of the same gender. That would unbalance the interview and leave the other partner marginalised.

The counsellor may be faced with individuals or couples with innumerable emotional difficulties in the prenatal area. A couple may deal with emotions differently and if either one has a minimising style there can be great emotional distance between them. Another problem is that the partners can have different views about testing the foetus or termination of the pregnancy. The counsellor may also find it difficult to maintain a neutral position if personal views conflict with those of the couple. When the partners deal differently with the upset of the situation, the most common situation is of the woman being more overtly emotionally upset, either crying or being angry, whilst the man does not display emotion so freely. The pitfall for the counsellor in working with difference between couples would be to try to bridge the gap, or to view the one as healthy and the other as the problematic. For example, emotional expression could be seen as healthy or open and therefore positive, whilst putting a negative construction on the less expressive way of being. Under that circumstance, rather than attempting to repair or improve the situation, it is more helpful to describe the difference between the two in a simple manner with a comment such as, 'I wonder if what we are seeing is the way you handle stressful and upsetting events differently as both of you are trying to come to terms with this situation'. This puts a positive construction on their different ways of dealing with the situation and often leads to a more open and compassionate discussion of their difference.

Another way of working with differences of emotional expression is to think systemically and see the difference as a balanced interaction. Comments such as the following can be useful, 'You are dealing with this difficulty in different ways and, although it looks as if there is a big difference between you, it seems to me that you may be helping one another. You x are expressing the upset for both of you; whilst you y, are attempting to find some control. So you are both making sure that there is a balance of upset and control'. Conversely, the counsellor could draw out the way in which the difference is maintained by the inter-relationship of their behaviour. So the more the one is upset, the more the other withdraws and vice versa. What then would happen if the one were not so upset, or the other not so withdrawn?

A further suggestion would be to explore their ability to comfort one another. This offers an opportunity to think about how intimate they are able to be. Directly asking, 'I wonder how you two are able to be close and comfort and support one another'. Inviting them to recall times when they were close can help the couple think about how they are, how they were and how they would like to be.

Examples

1. In the following example a counsellor recognises that the partners are separate and tries to bridge that gap with helpful suggestions, but it results in an angry retort.

   After an amniocentesis, a woman had a result which confirmed that the foetus had a genetic disorder and she wanted to have a more informed view of how the child might be affected. She came for the consultation with her sister, as her husband was working away. The counsellor gave the information and was interested in the absence of the husband. Imagining that he might want information, the counsellor offered to see him at another time, or to give the wife a letter with all the relevant information which she could give to her husband. The woman's reply was that she had told her husband there was a problem and she did not intend telling him anymore, as all he ever wanted was perfection.

The counsellor had sensed the husband's exclusion and helpfully tried to redress the balance. The intervention was rejected by the woman and, as a result, the counsellor was excluded. It is interesting that the counsellor, not knowing the nature of the relationship, senses something and empathises with the man who is absent and offers to help him. The counsellor was forced to personally experience that exclusion by the woman's sharp retort and was taken aback by the anger not knowing what to do or say. The pain of exclusion and the sense of not knowing what to do were countertransference experiences, forcing the counsellor to feel what it was like to be part of the family. The counsellor's thoughts about the absent husband were important and discussed in supervision. It was suggested that rather making a helpful offer, using the sensitivity of absence to ask questions around the experience might have produced a different response. The following questions were a few suggestions: the counsellor could explore what the husband might think if he were present, what difference would it make if he were told, how the couple had spoken about the problem or how they shared difficulties. However, given the sense of closure the woman introduced, it would not be surprising if most approaches proved to be unhelpful.

2. In this second example, a couple have had two previous pregnancies and both children had been affected with cystic fibrosis. The woman was pregnant again and there was the question of testing the present pregnancy. She did not want any intervention and pleaded with her partner not to make her go through it all again, saying that she would wait until the baby was born to know if the child had cystic fibrosis. He, however, wanted to know whether again they would have a child with cystic fibrosis, arguing that he needed time to adjust and prepare.

   The couple appeared very separate and the woman made comments about his lack of involvement but then, suddenly, she distanced him completely by telling him that this was not about him, but about her. That comment came as a surprise and it took a while for the counsellor to be able to think. Eventually, the counsellor made the comment that it seemed so difficult for them to find an agreement. Unfortunately, the interview did not result in an agreement being reached by the couple – the woman acquiesced as she could not continue to resist her husband's reasoning. The couple remained fixedly apart. When they received their result, which was that the foetus was affected, he became very upset and the same day she collapsed in the supermarket.

   Both partners were devastated by the result. The woman had been aware that it would be extremely difficult for her but the extent of the man's upset had not been predicted. In retrospect one possibility could be that their conflict distracted and protected them from grieving for what had already happened. Focusing on the previous pregnancies, their disappointments and fears might have facilitated more emotional processing. The woman in this example stated that she did not want to go through it all again and suggests that she was still traumatised by her previous experiences. The urgency for a decision and the intensity of the emotions make these interviews extremely difficult. When there is a distressing distance between a couple, counsellors can easily be seductively drawn into problem-solving. However, empathising and exploring what it all means can be more productive.

Huntington's disease

The long experience of working with Huntington's disease, both genetically and psychosocially, has resulted in the development of a service protocol (Craufurd and Tyler, 1992; Harper, 1997) and the experience has been extended and used as a template for the presymptomatic testing of other late-onset genetic disorders. The general format is that of a preliminary exploratory meeting followed by two further interviews, where particular aspects of the disorder and its implications are covered. The time between the interviews gives space for reflection on the decision to be tested and the implications for the individual and extended family. A further meeting is arranged for the test result and can be followed by a number of possible follow-up meetings. In a study assessing predictors of adjustment to testing for Huntington's disease, those less well-adjusted after testing positive were married, had no children, and were nearer the age of estimated age of onset of the disorder (Codori et al., 1997).

The following extract is from a first consultation after a preliminary interview. The counsellor explains the overall plan but the educative intervention also addresses and focuses on the implications for the individual.

'I just want to explain a little bit about what's going to happen, as there is quite a long procedure about finding out whether someone may or may not have Huntington's disease and the reason for that is that there are quite a lot of different things people have to think about, because it's sort of knowing about the future'. The counsellor continues and explains inheritance patterns before returning to the patient's particular circumstance, 'We are not sure what happened, whether your father had the faulty gene because he died at the age of 55 and didn't have any signs of Huntington's disease … and that makes it a little more likely that he had the normal one, but it doesn't necessarily follow, it's not absolute. But it does make the fifty–fifty chance go down. If he had the faulty gene then there would be a fifty–fifty chance but at the moment we don't know … and you don't have any brothers or sisters.… So that's how we get to 25% chance, one in four … but it's actually less because your father didn't have any signs at the age of 55 years … We can do a test on you and if you've got the gene then it still doesn't tell you when you will have problems'.

This is a very clear educative intervention which included the fact that people approach the decision to be tested for different reasons and that the decision requires time and thought. It would usually be followed by a more psychologically based approach which allows time for a reflective stance where the individual can address the personal meaning of being tested. The counsellor may facilitate increased awareness by inviting speculation or imaginary scenarios. For example 'Can you imagine receiving your result?' or 'How would you go about talking to your partner?' 'How would it be if you tested …?'

Any number of different family scenarios can arise and the following are three examples.

Examples

1. This extract is taken from a preliminary consultation of a couple where the woman, who has a family history of Huntington's disease, considers the possibility of testing in the context of her siblings having differing views on testing and pregnancy. Although she seems clear about being tested, the counsellor invites her and her partner to talk about their belief systems and prevailing moods.

   She had requested testing as they wanted a family. The woman revealed, 'I've seen my sister and she's had three kids, but wasn't tested until after the children were born and then I saw my brother and he had the embryo tested. I think I'd rather know before I start a family'. The counsellor responded, 'I guess you must have discussed what influence the result would have on you' and was given the reply, 'If I've got the gene, I'll do the same as my brother and have the embryo tested, … although it seems a bit callous, it does seem a good idea … knowing I'd be able to stop the gene'. The counsellor asks 'How much of your thinking time is taken up with Huntington's?' and the woman replied, 'I've grown up with it. Every time we go round my mother's, it's there and the subject comes up. But my Mum's brothers and sisters, really nobody talks about it, they walk away and one of them totally believes Huntington's disease doesn't exist'.

   The counsellor invited the couple to explore how anxious they felt and the woman answered, 'I'm was fine about this appointment … but then thinking I was starting to get nervous and think "what if I do have Huntington's disease?" We've talked about it a lot and he thinks I haven't got it, but I think I have'. The couple then reflected on other family characteristics which were influencing their suspicions and further acknowledged that they had been depressed recently, which the counsellor wisely construed as possibly preparing them in case they had bad news.

2. In this second example a woman explained she had been in hospital and the subject of her family history of Huntington's disease had come up with her physiotherapist who had said 'Why don't you find out?' At a later point in the interview it emerged that the woman had requested testing some time ago but her affected mother had refused to be involved. More recently, the problem had been bothering her as she had developed pins and needles in her leg and had headaches. She confessed that she associated every symptom she had to Huntington's disease and so now 'I want to be clear one way or another. If it's yes, then so be it and then you have to face the future and prepare the children. My son is a worrier, tell him and he'd be in the surgery the next morning'. The counsellor continued to explore the woman's experience of the disorder and learned that as a child she had been subjected to violence. That experience, together with personal fear of a change in personality, was triggering her desire to be tested in order to make adequate preparation for herself and inform her children.

The counsellor's task in this example was to listen to the woman's story. She was linking her past experience as a child of a parent suffering from Huntington's disease with her present motivation. Her intent was not to repeat the past, but to take responsibility by being tested and, if necessary, make preparations for her own care.

3. This is another example of a young couple requesting testing as they were planning a family but they had a particular dilemma. The husband had a family history of Huntington's disease on his father's side, but the father had not been tested and that created a dilemma for the couple. The couple struggled with this issue knowing the implications of how testing the husband could reveal the father's genetic status. The counsellor helped them think through their concern for the husband's father whilst also considering their future and that of a child. They were very clear that if the test confirmed the husband carried the mutation, they would not have children. They resolved their dilemma by deciding they would keep the result a secret from the father. The husband proceeded to be tested.

These examples illustrate some of the personal struggles which come into the genetic encounter. This is only the tip of the iceberg as such a small percentage of people at risk come for testing. Each individual who does not seek testing will have a personal story. Some may have decided to carry on living believing they are free of the mutation (consciously or unconsciously denying their vulnerability); some will be aware and too frightened; others may make unnecessary sacrifices in their lives based on the unconfirmed belief that they carry the mutation.

Cancer genetic clinics

The service planning for predictive testing in these clinics is based on the experience of working with Huntington's disease with the protocol consisting of a preliminary discussion followed by two interviews. In these interviews, standardised information is covered and relevant issues explored. A family history is taken early in the process and this clarifies the degree of risk from the genetic component. The information covers all aspects of the disorder including treatment or monitoring possibilities, potential problems in terms of insurance and mortgage and the implications for the individual and family. The second of the two interviews gives more space to personal reflection for the individual and, if the decision is to be tested, blood samples are taken at the end of both interviews. The result is given at an agreed time and, as will be seen in one of the examples, in some instances in an agreed way.

At one level the interviews in this clinic follow the general pattern of all genetic consultations, but there is a slightly different emphasis in that a family history of cancer has to be balanced against the occurrence of cancer in the general population. There is also the possibility of screening and monitoring which offer early detection of the disorder and treatment. This fact will influence not only the percentage uptake of testing but also will bring in a degree of hope. The educative intervention will be geared to clarify these points and highlights a marked difference between the interviews for cancer and Huntington's disease. The interventions however are not solely educative. In a recent survey of UK centres, which explored the practice for hereditary non-polyposis colorectal cancer, both educative and reflective counselling were used (Brain et al., 2003).

A study by Thewes et al. (2003) reported that in a small proportion of women with a family history of breast cancer there was a strong desire to participate in a group where they could learn more about cancer genetics and discuss feelings related to their family history. Karp et al. (1999) designed a programme of a six-session psycho-educational support group for women at high risk for breast cancer who were considering prophylactic mastectomy. They concluded that the group work was beneficial.

Most individuals perceive their risk of cancer as higher than it truly is. Sometimes this is a perception coloured by the personal experience of seeing relatives with the disease. Although by training the genetic counsellor wants to give precise numerical risk figures, Stadler and Mulvihill (1998) reported that patients were more likely to remember risk if the interpretation was understood as an increase, decrease, or no different from their pre-counselling perception. The authors also caution against counselling creating a barrier to surveillance by neither raising anxiety, nor giving a sense of false security where the risk is lower than expected. France et al. (1999) raised the importance of considering the affected, as well as the high-risk worried, as both need counselling information and follow-up.

The following extract gives an idea of the overall planning of an interview for predictive testing in cancer genetics.

Extract

C: Let me give you an idea of what we are going to do today. I want to hear from you, what questions you have, and what brought you here. I think that will probably lead us to talking about your family history. That will help us decide whether the cancer in your family is there because cancer is common, or because your family have a predisposition for cancer. I wonder if you know how common cancer is.
P: Very common.
P: Yes. If nothing else affects us, then one in three will develop cancer. So we have to think, is this due to chance, or is something happening in this family. But what alerts us to there being a genetic predisposition is if there are a lot of people who have developed cancer, a lot in one generation and if we see that it is in several generations and if young people have developed cancer.
P: I know it can affect my children as well, so that's why I came actually'.

In this extract the counsellor focuses and structures the interview pathway so the patient knows exactly what is going to happen and the patient explains her motivation. After drawing a family tree the interview continues.

C: Looking at families like yours over many years we would be more prone to thinking that there is something going on in the family because there is a particular pattern.

The counsellor then draws diagrams to explain genetic inheritance likening each person's chance of receiving the faulty information as fifty–fifty, the same as tossing a coin each time.

P: So what about my children, that's what's worrying me.
C: Let's take it one step at a time. If it hasn't come to you then it can't go to your children. If it has come to you then it's not inevitable that the children will have the faulty gene, each child will have a fifty–fifty chance.

P: That's all much better than I thought, it's not a hundred percent and I thought I would definitely have it.

C: Even if you have the faulty gene it does not mean that you will definitely have cancer.

The counsellor continues.

C: So we've talked through the family history and the fact that we have some information about your family and in the next however long. I want to talk through with you whether you want or don't want to go through with this sort of testing. I'll be telling you what testing means, why some people choose to go ahead and why some choose not to. I'll be going through the pro and cons of testing.

The next part of the interview focused on the practicalities of testing, the advantages of screening and monitoring to detect early changes, and the disadvantages or possible problems which may arise from insurance companies.

C: You may then want to take a break to think things through.

P: No, I know I want to go through with it because knowing is better than not knowing.

C: We can take the blood today and we would look at your genetic blueprint and compare it to what this other blueprint is in your family. We will be able to see whether there is a match or not. So we'll know whether you have the normal or the faulty gene and at any point you can put a stop on it, you are in charge.

The counsellor then prepares the patient for the future meeting when the result will be given.

C: Let's imagine you have come for the result. Will you have someone with you?

P: My husband will come, I guess.

C: What will you do? Will you just fit it into your busy day, or do you think it is better to allow some time afterwards rather than rushing off?

P: Well, there's my work and my husband's work but I suppose we ought to take our time and may go and have tea somewhere, just to let it sink in.

C: How do you think you want to be told? Do you want some pleasantries or do you want me to just say either, 'It's good news or it's bad news?'

P: Just say it straight.

This is a very carefully crafted interview where the counsellor systematically goes through clearly defined issues and the woman's concerns are dealt with in a logical educative manner. This sort of interview demystifies cancer and gives potential sufferers a sense of control. However, there will be individuals and families who will not be able to manage the process. Some will not be able to contain their anxiety and are terrified; others keep the family history secret.

Example

A woman, having been tested positive, was not prepared to continue with monitoring for breast and ovarian cancer, and decided that only with surgery could her anxiety be allayed. She had lived with her mother and aunts all of whom had cancer of the breast and seen the anguish it had caused. There had been no discussion or sharing of information or anxieties; the female members anxiously waited their turn and silently wondered who would be next.

Whilst genetic testing can offer hope in familial cancers if the testing is done presymptomatically, the genetic counsellor frequently has contact with family members who are dying and leaving young children behind. It is enormously painful for a mother, who is dying of breast cancer, to tell her teenage daughter of the genetic pattern in the family. The task is huge. The dying mother has to come to terms with her own death before she can speak to her daughter, who may already be grieving, knowing her mother's future. In such circumstances a family may have been depressed for many years. There is no easy answer and the genetic counsellor will need to be able to tolerate raw grief to sit alongside these anguished families.

Dysmorphology clinics

The problems in these clinics can be very varied but usually take the form of a diagnosis of an unusual-looking child. When there are associated disorders, the function of the diagnosis is clear and clarifies what specialist medical or educational help is needed. In contrast, where there are no associated problems, the function of the diagnosis is questionable and will be determined by an assessment of parental attitudes. The diagnosis can either act as a container of anxiety or, in contrast, it can be anxiety-provoking. In the former the diagnosis may make something which is thought of as unusual, understandable; in the latter, especially in sensitive or vulnerable families, the diagnosis can be perceived as very traumatic and seriously interfere with the parents' perception of the child. It is as if the child is changed in some way.

When a child is born looking different, odd, or disfigured, then the difficulty is initially the parents' who have to process their disappointment. The success or failure of that process will determine their perception of the child and, as a consequence, the parent/child relationship. Later on, the child will have to make the adjustments: to cope with being different, struggle with personal self-image, attempt to integrate and be accepted by the peer group.

Siblings may also be affected (Lansdown et al., 1991). Being different puts the child at risk of being teased but it is interesting to note that the relationship between facial deformity and psychological effect is not linear (McGregor, 1970). The mild, rather than severe deformity, is harder to cope with (Lansdown et al., 1991). A possible explanation could be that the more obvious deformity has to be acknowledged, whereas the nearly normal may stimulate the desire and anxiety to be accepted as normal. The subject is difficult to research as asking a child or a parent whether or not they are stared at, or how they cope with looking different is a sharp and potentially hurtful reminder of the problem. The reports of the existing studies are conflicting with self-esteem being reported as lower and also higher than normal. The latter is explained by the experience of having to cope with adversity (Brantley and Clifford, 1979). Bradbury (1993) considers that children and their parents show signs of stress, anxiety, depression and social isolation, which will have an effect on the dynamics of family life.

The birth of a child with a deformity is a uniquely traumatic event for the mother. During pregnancy the child is considered part of her and so a deformity in the child affects the mother's self-image. This can result in conscious and unconscious feelings of devaluation and worthlessness. The thoughts might include, 'What is wrong with me? Why has this happened to me? What have I done?' Lax (1972) has described the process as narcissistic trauma and Kohut (1971) describes how the baby is experienced as the defective part of the self. The counsellor's explanations are vital, even if no cause is known, as they serve the function of balancing the mother's sense of personal responsibility. Solnit and Stark (1962) have described the responses as mourning and Fajardo (1987) refers to the ambivalence experienced by parents who have grieved for the loss of the child they expected to have. In studies of parenting it has been proposed that the deformed face is more difficult to read (Field and Vegha-Lahr, 1984), with mothers showing less responsive smiling at 3 months. In contrast, Hoeksma and Koomen (1991) have reported that mothers are more inclined to over-stimulate babies who look unusual.

The parental attitude is a key factor in the initiation and maintenance of the child's self-image. The mother physically holds her infant in her arms; emotionally in her mind. A mother might try and pretend that the dysmorphology is of no consequence, but does not succeed in fooling the child who perceives what the mother thinks and whether the love is genuine or not. The mother's eyes are the mirror in which the child first views her or himself. As the child grows he/she will be able to recognise personal difference and will have to mourn the loss of personal normality. This is a painful process and yet necessary to promote autonomy and self-worth. Even the strongest motherly love will not be able to protect a child from the arrows of being looked at by society. A child may use numerous defensive-adaptation mechanisms to cope with being different. Timberlake (1985) grouped the defences as: erasure, symbolic repair and encapsulation. Erasure involves the child in pretending to be different as for example by having a magical cure of some kind. In symbolic repair the child collects things which are considered to make a difference or strives to be an expert in a specific area. Encapsulation involves the child in a lot of planning and sets things up in an attempt to control a situation.

The face is our contact with the world and expresses emotions, attitudes and even our hidden thoughts. We project ourselves outwards where we are read by others and in return we see ourselves in the facial response of others. How does facial deformity interrupt this process? In the past it has been explained by folklore and even in today's more enlightened society many misconceptions persist (Shaw, 1981). Fairy stories and mythology incorporate these early cultural beliefs with the disfigured face symbolising evil (Bradbury, 1993). The disfigured child is consistently placed at the bottom of ratings for preferences for companionship (Lansdown et al., 1990) and can be perceived as being less intelligent. Goffman (1963) held that facial deformity could stigmatise individuals, making them less acceptable to society. This may hold true today with our focus on image and the failure to accept even the natural changes of aging with the use and abuse of plastic surgery. We are indeed in the age of 'The Beauty Myth' (Wolf, 1990).

The counsellor's interventions in dysmorphology clinics are both educational and directed to facilitating emotional processing. The function of the diagnosis is crucial and there is particular need to assess the sensitivity of the parents and child. An example of the sensitivity of a parent to a child's diagnosis is given in the discussion of empathy requiring the use of tact as presented in Chapter 4. Timberlake (1985) recognises the significance of a diagnosis and has suggested that interventions should facilitate mourning and cognitive restructuring to help with internal representations.

This analysis of the four different genetic disorders has shown how the educational intervention is common to all but, in each disorder, it is slanted to take into account the significance of the disorder and the impact of a diagnosis or test result. Psychological interventions are also necessary and are again related to the particular disorder and the individual. Grieving and containment of anxiety are common to all disorders but each disorder triggers a particular psychic pain and necessitates the counsellor be sensitive to the difference. Where there are prenatal problems the counsellor is mindful that the educative information presented needs to give as accurate and objective view of the foetus as possible. This helps redress any misperceptions based on fear or denial, as it will be an important factor in the decision about the future of the pregnancy. In Huntington's disease the emphasis is on exploring the significance of the diagnosis and the motivation for testing in the context of personal resources. The educational intervention in cancer genetics takes into account the importance of monitoring and early treatment and demystifies the disorder by addressing the aura built up around the popular perception. A particularly delicate touch is needed when dealing with problems of dysmorphology, balancing the function of the diagnosis against the psychological impact on the parents and developing child.

Summary points

The pattern of the overall process of genetic counselling is not a straight line, but a series of spirals, where each circle is observing and auditing the last intervention. The result of this constant auditing means that the formulation of the meaning of the original question may be quite different from its initial appearance and, as a result, the consultation may take a winding path to its conclusion.

The nature of different genetically determined disorders will influence the consultation not only in content but also because each disorder has different implications and consequences, with different options open to the individual. The counsellor's sensitivity to the implications of the disorder determines how a consultation is focused and where there is a need for particular delicacy.

9

The effect on the counsellor

This chapter explores how working in medical genetics can be emotionally challenging for the counsellor and examines it under two broad headings: factors relating to the nature of the task and countertransference issues. The former relates to the fact that genetic counselling is inherently stressful and very painful for families and individuals. The latter refers to factors arising as a result of working with a particular individual, countertransference issues. The counsellor needs a diversity of the skills to work effectively to help and not be overwhelmed. This chapter will demonstrate how the counsellor's self-exploration can be personally beneficial and, if understood, it can enrich the overall encounter by adding another dimension of meaning to the behaviour of the patient and the interactional relationship. Regular supervision creates a safe psychological space for exploration and learning.

The nature of the genetic counselling task

The nature of the counsellor's task is complex and has been one of the main areas of interest in this book. At this point it is considered in relation to two areas: the particular skills mix required and the giving of 'bad news'.

The skills required

Working in the field of medical genetics brings many exciting opportunities to study a speciality in the forefront of scientific medicine whilst also being in touch with the human side of the work, talking and working with people. This is rewarding and affords the counsellor the opportunity to develop these seemingly different aspects of the self, the scientific and more emotionally-attuned. The role of the counsellor requires a mix of skills; sometimes it involves giving information and sometimes acting as a facilitator. These roles necessitate the counsellor moving in and out of being 'an expert'. 'The expert' is the information-giver who knows the genetic facts of inheritance patterns and the behaviour of particular genes in genetically determined diseases. The facilitator has questions, not answers and is a companion to a patient who is struggling to find a path through the emotional experience. In the former role, the professional is clear and has a strength which comes from that specific knowledge. In the latter, the professional is tentative with the strength coming from being able to tolerate 'not knowing' comfortably waiting, not in helplessness but, grounded in a quiet confidence and belief in autonomy.

Sometimes the counsellor splits these roles as consultations can have a different focus. At other times the counsellor needs to switch skills within one consultation. This means behaving differently and using different personal abilities. However, looking at transcripts of interviews, listening to reports of interviews and reading the letters written to patients after counselling, it is interesting and rewarding to see that it is possible. Nevertheless, it needs to be acknowledged that the counsellor is often more comfortable in the role of the informer (when the counsellor can use educative interventions). The counsellor's familiarity with this style can result in it being overused and adopted when emotional attunement might be more appropriate. In addition, the counsellor knows that information overload is unhelpful, but it is not easy to know how much information a particular individual needs. Giving too much information or staying in an educative mode may be triggered by the counsellor's anxiety to cover all aspects of the genetics in great detail and ensure the job has been well done. Alternatively, the strategy can be used to protect the counsellor from working with the patient's anxieties, or conceal an inexperience in the use of more extensive counselling skills. The ability to work with a patient's anxieties begins with the counsellor being personally aware and secure, specifically in the areas of anxiety and depression. In addition, integrating the emotional aspect of genetic counselling with information-giving necessitates an internal balancing of the intellectual and emotional aspects of the self. This personal, internal integration of seemingly conflicting aspects of the self is quite a task, but, if it can be achieved, it enables the counsellor to move from one mode of communication to another.

Giving 'bad news'

Information-giving in genetic counselling includes not only giving the individual general genetic information, but also the relevant information about the personal genetic potential for disease and explaining its impact on the individual's present state of health or future potential health. Both are central to the practice of genetic counselling but, because of the impact of the latter, it necessitates considerable thought. It could be said that finding a creative thinking space encapsulates the essence of genetic counselling. This is particularly relevant in predictive testing where a considerable amount of time is given to considering and reflecting on the desire to be tested, the individual's degree of readiness and their appreciation of the consequences. The term 'giving bad news' has been adopted and has been defined by Buckman (1992) as giving information which drastically and negatively alters an individual's view of the future. The earlier chapter on stress has explained that the response to information is not directly related to the information itself but is a factor of the inter-relationship of the disorder and the individual's perception of its meaning.

The counsellor prepares an ideal setting for giving news by following the general form of genetic counselling covering so many aspects of the individual's past and present and, during that process, develops a strong working alliance. The counsellor invites the individual to imagine having different results and this mental rehearsal prepares the individual for the event. However, there is always a difference between the imagined and the actual so that, even with considerable preparation, unexpected upset can still arise. The rehearsal is also emotionally preparing the counsellor, who is also working through anxieties of how the process will be experienced and managed.

No one wants to be the bringer of 'bad news'; we prefer to be pleasing people and that makes us happy and leaves a good feeling all around. In contrast, the bearer of 'bad news' is the messenger who carries the information which can change an individual's life and that can impact on the counsellor in a number of ways. The counsellor is the first to have the information. Naturally, the counsellor reflects on how it might impact on the individual and, in that process, the counsellor triggers a personal preparatory grieving, before giving the news to the patient (Quill and Townsend, 1991). In predictive testing the topic is often included in a genetic counselling interview with advance agreement about how the individual wants to be told, whether face to face and in what manner; for example straight to the point, without any preliminaries, or led gently into the test result. This also allows the counsellor to self-prepare.

All counsellors but, in particular, those who are inexperienced, are appropriately concerned about their ability to give the news in a sensitive manner. The worries are not only about how the patient might react, but also (as witnessing distress is upsetting), that the counsellor might find the process very distressing personally and fear breaking down inappropriately. Alternatively, the counsellor can be left feeling depressed, or even responsible for causing the upset or harming the patient. When receiving 'bad news' some individuals become angry and target the counsellor who may react to the hurt by becoming defensively aggressive.

Brewin (1991) stresses the importance of the professional's manner in giving 'bad news' and considers that being kind and sad, giving the news gravely, or with too much sympathy and compassion, can lower morale. He advocates that good practice of giving bad news is in keeping with modern counselling and consists of a conversation rather than a prepared speech. It involves paying attention to the individual's personal characteristics and perception of the impact of the news, but, most importantly, reading the individual's immediate response. Seeing a glazed look in the individual's eyes is a cue for the counsellor to pause to try and understand the shock reaction. After an acknowledgement of the upset, the counsellor can then continue giving information which the individual may be able to take in.

Buckman (1992) is in agreement about the importance of the dialogue, but also puts forward a six-step protocol: preparing of the setting, clarifying the individual's knowledge and desire, sharing information in small chunks, repeatedly checking the individual's understanding, responding to the feelings expressed, before finally planning and organising future contact.

The following example illustrates one of the ways a counsellor may be affected by a counselling session and how supervision can be helpful.

In a supervision discussion the counsellor revealed that an interview had been very upsetting and described the degree of tiredness experienced at the end of a home visit. In the supervision the counsellor explored a number of issues. Did the consultation have any personal significance? Had the content of the consultation been particularly disturbing? Was the grouping of the extended family frustrating, with tensions and conflicts triggered by the genetic problem? The space given to the counsellor to explore, ponder and reflect may not have revealed the reason for the tiredness, but the process was supportive to the counsellor, especially as colleagues reported similar experiences.

Countertransference issues

In its broadest sense countertransference refers to all the feelings arising in the counsellor as a result of working with a particular individual. Our humanity and compassion allow us to be emotionally connected with others and to share their joys and pains. The positive side of being affected is that it enables us to help; our humanity enables us to reach out to one another and emotionally share by our empathic and compassionate responsiveness. However, in the world of medical genetics there is a negative side to being affected. Counsellors are exposed to the experiences of their patients who may be shocked, overwhelmed with anxiety or fear, grieving or struggling with relationship difficulties and many other emotional challenges. The genetic counsellor is therefore exposed to an emotionally highly-charged environment which can be personally upsetting, challenging or even draining and stressful.

The exchange of information and the professional conversation around genetic counselling is a human encounter in the service of the patient but, the counsellor is also there as a real person. The experienced and secure counsellor will have little difficulty acknowledging personal reactions but, sometimes, the less experienced or insecure can regard their personal emotional reactions as a lack of professionalism which needs to be hidden or denied. All counsellors are at risk of being disturbed at some point or another and they may experience physical sensations or feelings. Headaches, tiredness, or being depleted or stressed are common physical complaints; depression, anxiety or feeling unexpectedly angry, common emotional reactions. These feelings and sensations are unpleasant but can be understood, alleviated or even prevented by a deeper understanding of the delicate, interactional processes by which individuals affect one another. This involves addressing countertransference issues. In contemporary psychoanalysis, the historical idea of the analyst as a blank screen has been dismissed and all modes of therapy and counselling prefer to create the inter-subjective shared space. In the same way, modern medicine has changed and recognises that, when doctors or nurses hide behind desks or white coats taking refuge in defensiveness, it can result in coldness towards patients and the professionals themselves can close down and become depressed. The professional position of defensively distancing emotions is no longer considered constructive in psychotherapy or medicine. The difficult tasks of medicine have to be done which means defences are adopted as a necessary personal protection. However, the professionals might find it helpful to understand more about themselves, what goes on between people and how to process and use the experience for their own good and that of the patient.

An analysis of the concept of countertransference not only helps the counsellor with their personal feelings, but also furnishes the counsellor with additional information about the patient which can be an effective therapeutic tool. The counsellor becomes like a human barometer, recording impressions, feelings and attitudes. The skill is in learning to develop the self as an instrument and then knowing how to use it.

The term countertransference comes from psychoanalysis where originally it was considered a hindrance and a resistance on the part of the analyst, whose own neurotic conflicts were seen as being awakened in response to the patient (Freud, 1937). Over time, the understanding has changed and the definition widened. Based on Heimann's (1950) description, it is now regarded as one of the most important tools for understanding the patient's unconscious. The term encompasses all those feelings aroused or evoked by the patient, whether arising from the counsellor's personal life, the patient's emotional condition, the way the patient handles upset or the dynamics set up in the professional relationship. In simple terms the counsellor will be debating internally, 'Is this something to do with me and my past?' or 'Is this feeling telling me something about the pain of this patient?' or 'Is this connected to the relationship pattern set up by this patient?' 'Is this feeling something the patient is denying?' These questions will be explored further and then applied to genetic counselling.

The counsellor understands the patient's subjective experience by the process of empathy internally saying, 'I am feeling the feelings of the patient but it is not my world, it belongs to the patient'. However, sometimes the connection between the counsellor and patient goes beyond empathy and then becomes a particular form of countertransference known as projective identification, a term derived from the theory of Melanie Klein (1952). To explain it, Gordon (1965) uses metaphorical language and differentiates between three mental mechanisms: identification, projection and projective identification. Identification is likened to ingestion, where the two people think they are similar; projection is thought of as the psychic equivalent of excretion, where one denies feelings and projects them into the other; and projective identification is described as fusion, where ownership of behaviours and feelings is confused. Another useful explanation is given by Tarnopolsky (1995) who considers three countertransference positions which are based on the quality and intensity of projective identification. They are described as empathy, complementarity and enactment. In empathy, the counsellor resonates with the patient and develops an intuitive understanding of the patient and their situation; in complementarity, the counsellor experiences something the patient disowns; in enactment, the counsellor performs what the patient disowns. The internal dialogue of the counsellor might therefore include, 'I am feeling something of the patient's pain by being in tune' or 'I am feeling rather angry and the only way I can make sense of the feeling is that the patient is denying it' or further, 'I'm behaving uncharacteristically, I wonder if the patient is disowning feelings, pushing strong feeling into me which are forcing me to act uncharacteristically'. These experiences furnish the counsellor with an additional understanding of the patient by the development of an internal dialogue which cultivates self-awareness and asks the question: 'What is it like to be with this person?' or 'What am I feeling, thinking or registering physically'. The counsellor can learn to translate these ideas of countertransference and apply or adapt them with the help of regular supervision.

The following breakdown simplifies and adapts countertransference ideas to genetic counselling. Countertransference can be considered under these headings:

(a) Feelings belonging to the counsellor, with the re-experiencing of a previous personal experience which has been triggered by the patient.

(b) Feelings belonging to the patient but experienced by the counsellor, ranging from empathy to projective identification.

(c) Feelings arising in response to the attachment style of communication of the patient.

(d) The angry attack on the counsellor.

(e) The counsellor's distress at witnessing inadequate care in the family.

Feelings belonging to the counsellor

Genetic counselling contains all the experiences of living which includes births, deaths, illness and pain in individuals (adults and children). The drama of life's experiences is brought into consultations reminding counsellors of their own similar life stories, the universality of vulnerability, personal good fortune or tragedies. Kessler (1992b) remarked that 'over and again … professionals are exposed to material which tends to re-open their own past and current wounds'. This is a challenge inviting the counsellor to privately investigate their own emotional processing of both past and present experiences of shock, grief, anxiety and painful family memories. The emotional pain may be recent and the wound particularly raw which can result in the counsellor acknowledging that it is not appropriate to be working in areas where they are being confronted with reminders of recent, incompletely processed pain. The triggering of old experiences can be an opportunity for the counsellor to develop a deeper understanding of a past event which can be viewed again from a more mature perspective. Alternatively, the revisiting can bring a resurgence of emotional pain with a repetition of old unhelpful habits of defensiveness and distancing. This may interfere with the counselling process and prevent an open exchange and exploration of experiences for the patient.

Sometimes a counsellor may feel that they know how an individual patient feels because they have experienced something similar in their personal life. This process is called identification with the patient. In addition the counsellor may perceive similarities between patients. Both these situations can lead the counsellor to conclude prematurely that they understand and so make inappropriate remarks or impose ideas, without attending to the subtle differences which make every individual unique. Kessler (1992a) has suggested that the counsellor remains interested and inquires about the patient's particular experience. In that way the individual's uniqueness is respected and empathy becomes accurate. Further he does not agree with personal experiences being shared, considering that the practice can lead to boundary problems. He differentiates between being *friendly* and *being a friend* to the patient.

Training in psychotherapy has as a prerequisite that the trainees have personal therapy and supervision and this has been extended to some counselling training. The function of personal therapy is not only to support the professional in facing and resolving personal emotional issues, but it is also a direct training experience of being counselled by, and learning from, an experienced professional. Supervision provides a relationship in which the counsellor can think and learn about practice and this is discussed further at the end of this chapter.

Feelings belonging to the patient but experienced by the counsellor

When two people are together and one is talking about their life and its pain the most common experience is empathy. This enables the counsellor to under-stand the patient's subjective experience, which has been conveyed in words, feelings, actions and gestures. The counsellor achieves that understanding by not only listening and feeling, but also imagining what it must be like; asking questions to clarify and confirm what the patient is actually feeling. Tarnopolsky (1995) describes empathy as the resonance between patient and therapist, 'the I-know–how-you-feel' response, with a warm feeling of together-ness. In an earlier chapter on the skills of psychotherapy, the importance of including an understanding of intent was emphasised as giving empathy its full therapeutic power. Consider the following two statements in response to a grieving patient. In the first the counsellor reflects to the patient, 'you are very sad and missing your husband'. In the second the counsellor includes a further understanding by saying, 'you are sad, missing your husband very much and, in your grieving, you are trying to come to terms with the loss of him'. The first reflects the feeling and the reason; the second goes further and conveys an understanding that the feeling is part of the process where there is an under-lying internal struggle to master the psychological process of grieving.

Empathy involves the human ability of understanding emotional pain and utilises the ability to use our imagination and put ourselves in someone else's shoes. The ability to do so depends on intuition, insight, personal experience and theoretical knowledge. Usually the empathic feeling is put into words, so making an emotional bridge between the counsellor and patient. Occasionally the empathic response may result in the counsellor feeling quite upset. In moderation this can be useful.

Example

A patient, fearing he might have inherited the family disorder of a severe form of Ehlers–Danlos syndrome, graphically described his mother's last weeks and days and spoke movingly about his own unbearable helplessness. The counsellor continued to listen and stay with the patient and, in response to the sadness of the situation, was moved to tears. The interview continued. Towards the end, the counsellor began to make concluding comments but was interrupted by the patient who remarked that he had found it helpful to see that the counsellor had been affected and upset. More importantly, he had leant that it was possible to move into, and out of, the upset. The counsellor had acted as a model, demonstrating that upset could be managed, not allowed to overwhelm and does not need to be dismissed.

Whose anger is it? Projective identification

In the following example the feeling experienced by the counsellor is not empathy and presents a clinical challenge.

Example

A young couple, who have a handicapped child, had their fears confirmed that the wife had the Huntington's disease gene mutation. At a subsequent clinic visit, when the family again came together, it was clear that the patient was beginning to show signs of the disease. The emotional feeling in the consultation was interesting: the couple were rather flat and seemed withdrawn; the counsellor was extremely angry. The counsellor felt the anger was very surprising and was beginning to interfere with his ability to think clearly during the interview.

Clearly the situation for the young family was very distressing. It created another problem because they already had a handicapped child. The disorder would not only impact on the woman as a symptom bearer, but also on the couple's relationship. In addition, the child would probably suffer a premature loss of one parent. It is understandable that the counsellor would feel saddened for the couple but the anger and its extent was a puzzle. One hypothesis to explain the anger would be that the counsellor was frustrated – the interview was rather flat, the couple unforthcoming and no rapport was established. Another hypothesis could be that the counsellor was about the same age as the patient, inviting identification with the patient and triggering a feeling of injustice at a young life destroyed. A further hypothesis was that the anger belonged to one or both partners, with the feelings being denied in the couple and projected into the counsellor (projective identification). Both partners had very good reason to feel angry: the one for having the disorder and the other who stood to lose the expected future and be left as carer of the partner and the handicapped child. However, the important issue is not to be able to define the mental mechanism, nor to get the correct hypothesis, rather, to be able to explore the feeling and have ideas about how to use the experience.

The counsellor was sufficiently experienced not to act out the anger but held it and tried to help the couple explore the meaning of the test result for them (and how they reacted to the shock). The counsellor did not ask 'Are you shocked?' which would have been a closed question that could have provoked a straight rejection but used questions such as, 'I'm wondering how much of a shock this is to you both' and 'Which of you is most upset?' The latter approach is more likely to open an emotional discussion. It starts from an assumption that there would be some degree of shock and upset and invites them to not only explore their own feelings, but also to wonder about their partner. Other statements the counsellor might use include, 'I guess you are feeling a real mixture of feelings, try putting some of them into words'. However, these questions do not address the counsellor's anger. If the feeling is projective identification, the task is to help the couple reclaim the projected feeling. The following example is one way of working with the couple's lack of expression.

The counsellor might begin, 'You are both very quiet, I'm wondering if that is how you are normally, or whether this is your reaction to the news? Sometimes being quiet, when there is a lot of upset, is the same as putting a lid on something which is boiling up. If that's so for you, what feeling do you think might spill over? Would it be sadness or anger, or both?'

These suggestions are different ways in which the counsellor could explore the general hypothesis that the couple are projecting feelings and are gentle attempts to help the couple speak and claim their upset.

One of the most difficult clinical challenges is working with denial of feelings. It can frustrate the counsellor and the counsellor could easily become irritated, acting out the denied feeling. In the example described, the personal secure attachment pattern enabled the counsellor to hold and reflect on the projected feelings.

The effect of different attachment patterns on the counsellor

Attachment patterns evoke feelings in others and the nature of the different patterns will evoke a complementary response in the counsellor. No matter how difficult the issues discussed, when working with a securely attached person the counsellor is left feeling that the genetic interview went well, communication was easily established and it was relatively easy to attune to the patient and establish a two-way dialogue. This type of clinical experience is fulfiling and leads to a sense of professional satisfaction and the patient is appreciative of the care given. In contrast, insecure adults, having suffered some early assault on their capacity to develop relationships, bring their insecure representational models into the therapeutic relationship in vivid and immediate ways. The process of bringing relationship patterns alive in the consultation forms the basis of the counsellor's countertransference reactions (Slade, 1999).

Individuals with a dismissive style of dealing with life will minimise or ignore significant events and emotions. They may appear cold and distant, shutting out the counsellor, or they may be reactive and defensively brittle and appear to fight every idea discussed. Such an interview can feel barren, with no meaningful exchange. The counsellor is then left feeling that it was not possible to get through to the patient, as if a door had been closed. The seeming rejection of help can trigger feelings of frustration, hopelessness and professional impotence in the counsellor. One way of understanding this is that the patient is unconsciously forcing his early experiences (which can not be spoken) onto the counsellor, who then feels the anger and the sensation of being ignored, just as the patient had in childhood. This explains how there can be a recreation and a re-enactment in the present of an earlier interaction, as if the patient were saying, 'I can't tell you how things have been for me but I can make you do feel as I did?'

Another reaction in the clinician would be to try harder to engage the patient. That may result in the clinician becoming more forceful, creating a situation of escalating friction – a dynamic which may well be familiar to the patient. Alternatively, the frustration can lead to over-intrusion which invites further rebuff, leaving the counsellor hurt and possibly wanting to withdraw. The challenge here is how not to react by pushing harder in order to try 'and get through' and not to try and 'get inside'. Increasing the pressure on the patient will only result in an increased resistance. In contrast, asking a question about how previous difficulties have been coped with can sometimes result in the patient being more open and reflective. A long-standing pattern of having to manage alone is often revealed. Alternatively, commenting to the patient that it is difficult to know what to do with an upsetting or challenging situation can often free the resistance. This empathises with the difficulty and describes it, instead of reacting to it. These situations are very frustrating and the counsellor will find it helpful to understand the origins of the dismissive pattern. The patient's minimising style has arisen as a result of being unsupported as a child. Holding this idea in mind allows the counsellor to be more sympathetic and less reactive.

The other insecure pattern of attachment, the preoccupied, creates a completely different 'feel'. The consultation is coloured by the extremes of emotion, agitation, pre-occupation with the upset, a difficulty in calming down and an inability to tell a coherent story. In contrast to the rejection of comfort in a dismissive pattern, there is a hunger for comfort which is sometimes difficult to satisfy. The counsellor may feel overwhelmed or devoured by the patient's emotions and demands and may feel frustrated that no matter how much help or support is offered, it is not enough. The temptation is to fall into the trap of being impatient, which again the patient will have experienced before and thus will trigger further upset. The counsellor's natural response maybe to try and organise, but this is unhelpful. Empathising with the fact that the patient seems overwhelmed and that it is difficult to know how to soothe, can be containing for the patient. This intervention is addressing the process and the difficulty rather than the actual upset. Further, compassionately addressing how very upset the patient is and wondering what usually helps invites the individual to reflect on past experiences, to understand their usual reaction and to realise that the upset will pass.

Using a metaphor can also be a very simple and concise way of conveying an understanding. Expressions such as 'it seems as if the rug has been pulled from under you' or 'your world has been turned upside down' are immediately understood. A more direct approach is to ask a question which explores characteristic behaviour, 'I wonder what usually happens at home, how do you comfort one another or ask for comfort?' This is not only exploratory but also prescriptive, suggesting the need for comfort. The question also legitimises the patient asking for comfort.

It is extremely difficult to provide a secure base for reflection and to enter into the experience of patients who have an insecure attachment pattern and the attachment pattern of the counsellor plays an important part. Feelings flow from the counsellor to the patient as well as from the patient to the counsellor. With a secure pattern the counsellor creates an atmosphere of safety and connection. Making the consultation space a secure base is more difficult for a counsellor with an insecure attachment pattern and the counsellor is more vulnerable to being caught up in countertransference (Slade,

1999). However, on occasions, even counsellors with secure attachment patterns can fail to establish an emotional rapport.

The following example illustrates counsellors with secure attachment patterns being rejected by a couple with a dismissive pattern.

Example

A counsellor responded to a request to see a couple who had recently been told by a paediatrician that their child's developmental difficulties were the result of chromosomal problems. The couple were given the relevant information about the developmental problem of their child but, although it was pointed out that it was impossible to be more certain, they persisted in their request for a more detailed life course for their child. The counsellor was struck by the fact that the consultation lacked any emotion; there was no personal reference to the child but an emphasis on the syndrome. The atmosphere during the consultation remained brittle and tense in spite of the compassionate and considerate approach of the counsellor; the consultation was ended by the couple asking to see another counsellor. This was arranged but the first counsellor was left feeling frustrated and sad carrying in his mind a desire or a wish that the parents would show some personal sadness and affection for the child.

The second counsellor was met by the same unemotional attitude and a request for further testing and information about a centre with a particular interest in their child's disorder. A key issue in this consultation was the testing of the parents to explore the possibility of a chromosomal imbalance which might affect future pregnancies. The couple wanted the test done urgently which the counsellor organised and they were assured that, although the process would take some time, the counsellor would follow the process and make sure that everything was being done as quickly as possible. Again the second counsellor was left feeling that his best efforts had been dismissed.

The couple were subsequently given an appointment where they could be given their results – they cancelled and did not attend an arranged second appointment. This puzzled both counsellors. The two different counsellors had similar experiences and responses. Both were moved by the couple's situation, distressed at the lack of awareness of the child, concerned that the couple showed no emotion and disappointed that neither could establish a satisfactory relationship with the parents.

These consultations were conducted by very experienced counsellors who are secure in their practice and personally. As a result, neither fell into the trap of reacting to the couple's style by acting out their frustration. They remained patiently trying to help by always answering requests for more information and researching other centres where there was a particular interest in their child's condition. Unfortunately, neither counsellor succeeded in linking with the couple to help them and, like the couple, they were left feeling frustrated and dissatisfied.

The formulation of both counsellors was that the couple had an insecure and dismissive attachment pattern and were experiencing difficulty processing their grief which was denied in their unrelenting intellectual defence mechanism.

The sadness experienced by the counsellors was not empathy but projective identification so feeling the pain the couple were denying. The important question is 'How to work with the difficulty?' Both counsellors had used educative interventions and been extremely helpful and considerate but it would be interesting to speculate how they might use emotional interventions.

A direct emotional intervention based on empathy would be rejected by dismissive individuals. However, the intervention can be directed at the coping mechanism. For example, a positive construction of their way of coping would be to say, 'I can see how concerned you are by this news and clearly you want to really understand everything about your child's condition. In your search to understand and get the best possible care you are leaving no stone unturned. I applaud your search to understand everything in such detail, but I'm wondering how you are dealing with this problem and your comfort and support?' This statement joins with them by understanding their style of coping and then moves to concern for them.

Another approach would be to address the dynamic between the couple and the counsellor who, using the countertransference, might say something like, 'We've spent some time talking together, but I have a suspicion that you feel I'm not quite giving you what you want or need. I appreciate that there may be so much pain at the moment that nothing can help but help me understand what more I can do?'

There may be no way of helping some people and the counsellor has to live with the sadness of such situations.

The angry attack on the counsellor

An angry patient is always a challenge for the counsellor. There are times when the patient is justified in their anger, as for instance when kept waiting without an explanation. This is not a common occurrence as genetic counsellors are very aware of treating their patients with respect and consideration and have time-keeping as a priority. Occasionally, a counsellor may annoy a patient by making a mistake, but with appropriate apologies the damage can be repaired. However, sometimes the anger is inappropriate, disproportional or is the prevailing mood of the patient. When the anger is directed at the counsellor it can be very unpleasant, shocking and potentially destabilising. The counsellor may then take a defensive position and that invariably leads to further anger and the sequence is repeated. The angry attack may mean many different things, some of which include: uncontained emotions of an insecurely attached individual, a defence against pain, part of a grieving process or the result of personality difficulties. If at any point the anger becomes excessive or potentially dangerous then obviously the consultation will need to be closed, but fortunately that rarely happens.

The counsellor needs to be able to soothe or steady their own personal reaction and find an internal secure place. From that place it is possible to think about the patient's anger and not react to it. Inviting the patient to explain, 'Help me understand what's upsetting you?' is a good beginning. The answer may enable the counsellor to put a positive construction on the anger by describing it as 'helping with the distress' which can have a neutralising effect.

Alternatively, the following statement might be useful, 'I don't seem to be able to understand fully and we seem to be a bit stuck. We are trying to understand one another, but somehow I am not succeeding'. In both sentences the counsellor is taking a 'one down' position of not knowing, not reacting defensively, which could escalate to a disagreement. In other words, not joining with the sentiment but neutralising it.

In the next example the counsellor 'mops up' a couple's anger by a steady patient manner of explaining. Explanations are frequently used in genetic counselling and the invitation to the genetic counsellor in this book has been to be aware of other counselling techniques especially listening and relating. In this example the use of an educative intervention brings about an emotional change. However, it raises the question of the nature of the transforming agent. Was it the intervention, or was it the counsellor's patient and kind manner? Each time the patient expressed anger, the counsellor comes back with patience and good will.

Example

A genetic counsellor responded to a request for testing for Huntington's disease on a young boy of 10 years by making a preliminary home visit. The child's mother was seen alone and revealed that she was divorced from the child's father who had a family history of Huntington's disease. She did not know whether her ex-husband had been tested but two of his siblings had tested positive. Her second husband had expressed a wish to adopt her child but, before doing so, he wanted to know the child's genetic status. The visit went well with discussions around the inheritance pattern and the complexities of childhood testing.

At a subsequent clinic visit, the original counsellor was joined by a colleague. Both counsellors were surprised at the angry entry of the couple when the home visit had seemed to go well. Their demand was for the boy to be tested and their anger seemed to stem from their belief that they were being denied their rights. The counsellors explained the situation, but the couple continued to be angry and to such a degree that it could easily have destabilised less experienced or less robust counsellors. Although both counsellors were upset by the anger, neither reacted to it – rather, they remained patiently holding a quiet and clear position of information-giving and explanation.

The counsellor explained the situation was extremely complex and subtle, involving a highly personal and delicate issue, where there would be no immediate benefits of treatment or monitoring. Further, those decisions needed to be made by someone old enough to understand the consequences. Concern was expressed that the knowledge might interfere with relationships and the boy's development; the information would need to be carried for a long period of time and on reaching adulthood the child might view the testing negatively. At no point did the counsellor give a categorical yes or no but simply laid the current thinking before the couple. As the interview progressed the anger in the room subsided and the couple became more thoughtful. They were left to ponder further.

The counsellor used a number of interesting techniques: putting a positive connotation on their desire to know and plan; reframing the anger as a desire to do their best for the child; taking the patient out of their personal world, into the world at large and presenting a general viewpoint which reflected on the breadth of experience of the genetic community.

This has not answered the question of what was the transforming agent that settled the anger in this family. Was it the explanations, or was it the manner in which it was delivered? Certainly the information was an essential educative intervention. However, it was given gently, yet with authority, 'Let me try and tell you more about the thinking which has built up over many years'. In addition the pace of the interview was kept steady and not allowed to escalate in response to the repeated resurgences of anger. With explanations and by not reacting, the counsellors were absorbing the anger, digesting it and responding courteously with straight information. The counsellors did not react to the countertransference feeling of being shocked and taken aback (and possibly angry), but responded with a gentle explanation that neutralised the anger. The intervention was both educative and emotional. The technique of simply giving information may not have worked on its own. However, given the particular manner of quiet patient understanding by obviously experienced counsellors, the negative emotions expressed by the couple were transformed. The theoretical explanation for this transformation is based on Bion's work, described in Chapter 4. It refers to the ability to withstand the attack of negative emotions, internally process them and give them back in a different form. That process triggers the development of a mind and an ability to think and consider.

Witnessing inadequate care or painful family exchanges

Very often the genetic counsellor is moved by the loving support couples and families give one another. Equally, the counsellor not only hears stories of family distress, disharmony and trauma, but also witnesses in the consulting room emotional deprivation of couples unable to support or understand and comfort. Families may not only have to provide care for the affected family member but, because of the nature of the disorder, there may be a considerable amount of conflict, disharmony or even abuse. One of the most painful scenes is a parents' inability to provide adequate emotional care for their children. For example, in a group supervision discussion a counsellor spoke of her sadness and frustration at being unable to protect a child from witnessing a mother being scanned for a foetal abnormality (the counsellor's reasonable suggestions of alternative care for the child were overridden by the mother). Other distressing experiences include seeing a child pushed into premature adulthood by the needs of a sick parent. Alternatively, a parent may be emotionally immature and unable to offer reliability, forcing the child out of dependency into a 'pseudo-independence'.

Supervision

Exploring both the nature of genetic counselling and the emotionally challenging scenarios involved, confirms the importance of supervision in the counsellor's practice. It provides a secure place where the counsellor can do more than discharge emotions in what is frequently called 'off-loading'. Supervision provides support and a place for reflection and facilitates professional development. The understanding of the professional encounter can help the counsellor to deepen their own personal understanding and to increase the confidence to enter dark areas, to tolerate anxiety and, by so doing becomes stronger.

In every day usage the term supervision means a process of overseeing, evaluating and advising. In the counselling and mental health world the term refers to the process of consulting with another professional or group experienced in the area to create a thinking space. The supervisor or group establish a secure-enough base where the counsellor can process and reflect on the patient, the personal reactions and the counselling relationship. 'Supervision thus provides a container that holds the helping profession in a "therapeutic triad"' (Hawkins and Shohet, 1989). Similarly Kennedy (2000a) uses the Winnicott metaphors of the 'holding environment' and the 'good-enough mother' (1965, 1971) to think about supervision.

Supervision is a central and essential part of training and in general counselling it continues as part of on-going practice, even for the most experienced counsellors. Although the material for this book has arisen out of a supervision group for genetic counsellors, the existence of such a group is unusual as it does not, as yet, have such a central place in the profession as a whole. Kessler (2000) has asked important questions about the standards and skills for supervisors and wonders about the requirement to obtain supervision being set more stringently. He sees supervision as a matter of survival for the profession, as well as of vital importance for personal growth. He recognises that some people may not like being supervised as it can be anxiety-provoking but, encouragingly, he highlights the importance of over-coming obstacles.

The counsellor may be prevented from taking advantage of supervision by cultural or financial blocks at an organisational or personal level. The counsellor may need to be seen in a good light or as competent and may fear being exposed as inadequate. For supervision to exist there has to be a desire to understand, learn and make progress individually and organisationally. Supervision offers a supportive relationship where the clinical work is to be explored and anxieties acknowledged rather than criticised. The counsellor's attachment style will also influence the attitude to supervision. If it is insecure/dismissive it may result in the significance of supervision being denied, or there may be a difficulty in receiving from others. When there is an insecure preoccupied attachment, the counsellor may have difficulty feeling held and safe and in recognising that the experience is good-enough.

The supervision space can be seen as mirroring or paralleling a counselling session and needs a corresponding clear framework of confidentiality and safety, where anxiety can be acknowledged, questions asked, new ideas developed, self-awareness increased and new perspectives on technique and style gained (Kennedy, 2000b). Mollon (1997) highlights the importance of the relationship between the supervisor and counsellor and describes the process as a journey of discovery in which the two together reach a goal, or find the unexpected, whilst Weil (2000) considers that the connection to supervision helps with feelings of isolation and the desire for support.

Ideally the supervisor and line manager should not be the same person, but there is nevertheless a managerial aspect to supervision which is related to quality control ensuring that the standard of work is appropriate and ethically sound. It has two other components; educative, which may be direct teaching or a reflection on the work which is presented in order to improve skills and supportive, to ensure that the counsellor is not left to carry worries or work loads inappropriately but at the same time can understand the meaning of any anxieties raised (Hawkins and Shohet, 1989).

There are three basic types of supervision: individual (Kessler, 2000), peer group (Likhite, 2000; Bosco, 2000) and leader-led group (Kennedy, 2000b; Hiller and Rosenfield, 2000). There are advantages and disadvantages to all these types. Individual supervision offers privacy and personal experience but that has to be balanced against the multiplicity of perspectives and support from a group (Counselman and Gumpert, 1993). There are some worries that a group may become too supportive and lose the challenge to develop (Kessler, 2000) added to which the individual has the opportunity to present work only once in a period (Counselman and Gumpert, 1993). In addition some counsellors feel shame or embarrassment in sharing their work (Kennedy, 2000b). However, a group has the potential to modulate this vulnerability by seeing others making mistakes and learning within a supportive safe environment. Recognising the human capacity for self-delusion, Kessler (2000) prefers to work with audio- or videotapes or verbatim transcripts of a counselling session.

The focus in supervision will depend on the style of working, the setting and the experience of the counsellor. Whether the supervisor adopts a teaching or explorative stance, there is always the opportunity to model a thoughtful and reflective attitude. Hawkins and Shohet (1989) describe six modes of supervision but recognise that good supervision involves movement from one mode to another as appropriate:

1. Reflection on the content of the clinical session.
2. Exploration of the strategies made by the counsellor.
3. Exploration of the therapy process and the dynamic of the counselling relationship.
4. Focusing on the counsellor's countertransference.
5. Focusing on the here and now experience of the supervision session as a mirroring of the counselling session.
6. Focusing on the supervisor's countertransference.

Sometimes in supervision a situation is reframed and a new more constructive meaning is given to the same situation.

Supervision is about the counsellor learning, developing, being looked after and personally thinking about self-caring. The process can be a very enriching experience. Nevertheless, it can expose areas which need to be taken to individual counselling or therapy and a boundary between supervision and personal counselling needs to be established. A counsellor who has confronted the personal shadow of depression and recognised internal anxieties and vulnerability is more likely to be able to be a companion to patients who bring the darkness of despair and their many faces of distress. Counselling is therefore not based solely on techniques which have been learned. Techniques are important but they have to be integrated with a personal internal security and compassion for others.

Personal counselling or therapy is not the only path for personal development. The counsellor can also find a personal balance in relationships, sport, art, music and many other stimulating and relaxing pastimes and pleasures. A lot of these experiences are totally absorbing and therefore have the effect of stilling the mind and putting anxieties in perspective. This experience is described by runners, musicians, artists and many others who are totally engrossed in what they are doing. A more formal approach to stilling the mind would be to learn a meditative technique of mindfulness. This technique trains the mind to be in the moment, allowing intrusive thoughts to fall away. Such a skill has the additional effect of centring and grounding the individual and that can help in extremely stressful situations. These different life experiences are not meant to be dustbins for unpleasant emotional experiences or distractions from worries but are addition ways of personal growth and development.

Summary points

Working in clinical genetics is emotionally challenging as a result of its inherently stressful nature which requires a complex skills mix and counter-transference issues.

Sometimes it involves giving 'bad news' and seeing people very distressed.

The term countertransference encompasses all those feelings aroused or evoked by the patient, whether arising from the counsellor's personal life, the patient's emotional condition, the way the patient handles upset or the dynamics setup in the professional relationship. In simple terms the counsellor will be debating internally, 'Is this something to do with me and my past?' or 'Is this feeling telling me something about the pain of this patient?' or 'Is this connected to the relationship pattern triggered by this patient?'

Countertransference can be used as a tool as it enables the counsellor to understand more about the patient. It can be adapted and applied to genetic counselling under these headings:

(a) Feelings belonging to the counsellor, with the re-experiencing of a previous personal experience which has been triggered by the patient.

(b) Feelings belonging to the patient, but experienced by the counsellor ranging from empathy to projective identification.

(c) Feelings arising in response to the attachment style of communication of the patient.

(d) The angry attack on the counsellor.

(e) The counsellor's distress at witnessing inadequate care in the family.

Supervision can be a resource for the counsellor both personally and professionally by being a secure-enough base where the counsellor can process and reflect on the patient, the personal reactions and the counselling relationship.

10

The interview and non-directiveness

Debating the possibility of non-directiveness

The earlier chapters have presented a theoretical underpinning for genetic counselling (stress), a framework for understanding differences in individual behaviour (attachment theory) and various micro-skills (empathy, etc.) to furnish the counsellor with an appropriate repertoire. This final chapter returns to looking at the overall picture, using a wide-angled lens to explore 'the culture' of genetic counselling. The terms genetic counselling and non-directiveness have become synonymous and seem to be intertwined in spite of the efforts of a number of authors to disentangle them and clarify meanings. Clarke (1991) has debated the possibility of achieving non-directiveness and further, whether it is desirable. Wolff and Jung (1995) consider that the demarcation from eugenics, the training of counsellors specifically for genetics and the infiltration of psychological counselling concepts have contributed to the idea of respect for patient autonomy in genetic counselling. They propose the term non-directive be dropped and that a more psychotherapeutic approach of exploring meaning and personal significance is more appropriate. Expressing a similar sentiment Weil (2003) considers that the term non-directive is a historic relic and an impediment to creative theory and practice. He proposes that the relevant components of balanced information without the counsellor imposing values be retained and that the central ethos should be to bring the psychosocial into every aspect of the work. In addition, there may be a difference in the counsellor's and patient's perception of the neutrality of the counsellor (Shiloh and Saxe, 1989). Kessler (1992a, 1997) has considered the terms 'directiveness', coercion and 'non-directiveness' and rightly states that it is difficult to know what actually takes place in consultations. His belief is that the terms directiveness and non-directiveness are not polar opposites, as there are similarities between the approaches in that both are counselling strategies which attempt to exert an influence. The former strategy is directed towards behaviour; the latter towards the patient's thinking. He considers that non-directiveness is more than withholding advice, rather it is an active process and involves a way of interacting and working with clients that aims to raise their self-esteem and leave them in control of their lives and decisions. He defines non-directiveness as 'procedures aimed at promoting the autonomy and self-directiveness of the client' and concludes that 'non-directiveness is possible but that it requires good counselling skills'.

The term non-directive counselling has been adopted from Carl Roger's Non-Directive counselling (Rogers, 1957) and is used to underpin genetic counselling. Rogers himself found the term non-directiveness was misunderstood and confused with passivity and he changed the title to Person-Centred therapy. Person-Centred therapy arose in reaction to the paternalistic approach of interpretive psychoanalysis, redirecting the focus to the desires of the client and placing personal autonomy or self-actualisation as its goal. This immediately conveys his belief that in therapy the client is the expert on his or her life and has the potential to grow and develop and realise their full potential. The counsellor is the learner, constantly listening to try and understand the client's story. The same pathway away from paternalism can be traced in medicine as it has moved to patient autonomy, an ideal which genetic counselling champions. There is an endless debate about the possibility of non-directiveness, even within Person-Centred therapy. However, there is an agreement that it is an ideal and an attitude. Further, the therapy is seen as a process of exploration of feelings and attitudes related to the problem areas in the patient's life, followed by increased insight and self-understanding. To facilitate the process Rogers considered that three core therapist characteristics were essential for success and states that they all have to be present: genuineness or congruence, unconditional positive regard and empathic understanding.

It is important to remember that the aims of genetic counselling are different from those of Person-Centred therapy. In the former, autonomous decision-making is the goal which is focused on and specific to medical genetics; in the latter, there is a wish to encourage a global experience of self-exploration and personal endorsement, leading to self-actualisation. As a result, the interview processes can be very different and require the counsellor to behave quite differently. Nevertheless, as far as genetic counselling is concerned, the counsellor would do well to adopt the principles of Person-Centred therapy. In particular, it may well be that it is the attitude of non-directiveness that genetic counselling needs to take from Person-Centred therapy.

In genetic counselling, the motivation to adopt non-directiveness has been an attempt not to influence the patient's decisions. Unfortunately, sometimes this has led the counsellor to adopt a defensive position of non-involvement, passivity, or defensive avoidance when under pressure, rather than a stance of engaged neutrality.

The struggle to remain non-directive is epitomised in the dilemma created when a counsellor is asked directly for a personal opinion, as for instance in the question 'What would you do?' The counsellor can be thrown off balance if working from the belief that the only answer to this question is to give a direct answer. Fearful of influencing decisions, the counsellor may give a defensive, or even rejecting, answer. However, if the counsellor has the idea that the thought behind the question needs to be understood, then the anxiety of answering might lessen. Starting from a position of using counselling skills as advised by Kessler (1992b, 1997), the first step would be to listen to the statement behind the question. In this instance that could be 'I'm confused and frightened and don't know what to do'. In that way the question is converted into a statement of anxiety which will then enable the counsellor to make a second step of responding in many different ways. The counsellor might respond with the following empathic statement, 'I can understand you wishing there was a clear, right answer and that I had that knowledge. But, unfortunately, there isn't a right answer. If there were, I would give it to you'. This statement is more than empathy as it contains the desire to help and also the impossibility of knowing what is right. Alternatively, the counsellor could explore the effect of getting an answer to the question and might say, 'I could tell you what I might do, but I'm not sure that would help you make your decision and I would worry that it might not be right for you'. Or, similarly, 'How do you think that might pan out if I told you what I would do? Would you follow me? And would that be right for you? What difference would it make, would it make it easier or more difficult for you?'

Another possible answer might be for the counsellor to say, 'I'd do much the same as you – struggle and get confused and struggle a bit more, until I was a bit clearer and all the time wishing someone would give me the right answer'. The last idea is in keeping with those of Kessler (1997) who proposed providing a framework for thinking to give the patient a path to follow. He also highlights that such requests are made in the context of the professional relationship, with the patient possibly not being given enough help and looking for more. Such an approach would lead the counsellor to comment, 'I wonder whether you are telling me that you would like more help from me in this dilemma?' Kessler further advocates that it is possible for the counsellor to make suggestions, but tentatively, leaving space for the individual to disagree.

Exploring a similar dilemma, both Kessler (1997) and Wolff and Jung (1995) debate the responses made by a counsellor when confronted by a couple who have differing opinions on what to do about a pregnancy in which trisomy was found (based on Fraser, 1979). They subsequently asked the counsellor 'What would you do?' and received an answer which included the statement of, 'Well, it's not my problem'. Both authors agree that the response was not in the spirit of non-directiveness and that the response dismissed the plea. They include in their suggestions a more therapeutic response involving the use of an empathic approach, exploration and clarification of some of the statements made by each one of the couple and an acknowledgement of the conflict between them.

Another approach, following the pattern of the last example, would be to listen first of all for the meaning of the question. Understanding the emotion behind the request, the counsellor might venture, 'I guess when the dilemma is very difficult, it can be frightening and confusing and I can understand the wish for someone else to sort it all out'.

Further, a systemic perspective would include understanding that the couple are reflecting different aspects of the dilemma; the woman feeling one thing and the man the opposite, a sort of splitting of the internal debate. This could lead to the counsellor putting a positive reframe on the difference between them by commenting, 'You are both working very hard to resolve this dilemma and are putting forward different ways of looking at the difficulty, making sure that all the different ways of dealing with this difficulty are considered'. Further, as in the last example, the counsellor could explore what difference it would make to give a personal opinion. Using a more classic psychoanalytical approach of exploring the relationship between the patient and counsellor, the following statement might be useful, 'I can understand how, when the going is tough and you can't yet agree, you turn to me hoping I can provide the answer, hoping perhaps that there is a right answer. It's disappointing there is no right answer but let's see if we can understand your different view points'.

The suggested responses to the question in both examples stay within the counselling frame of exploring the thinking behind the question, the use of empathy, wondering about the effect of an answer and the thinking about the meaning of the question in the context of the professional relationship. None give a personal opinion, but neither do they move away from the dilemma. Rather, the counselling skills enable the counsellor to move closer to the patient's thinking in a compassionate way, constantly trying to understand further, offering help through professional intimacy. In this way the counsellor can stay within the non-directive approach without becoming defensive or passive.

Rather than continue the debate about non-directiveness, it may be more helpful to acknowledge that we do influence one another and learn more about that and ask what is helpful and what is unhelpful. If we acknowledge that influencing is inevitable, then what is it that we would want to affect? Clearly it would be important to influence the way decisions are made. Shiloh (1996) has emphasised the importance of ensuring a decision is made wisely. In this book the approach taken is one of ensuring there is a theoretical base of understanding genetic counselling. In addition, identifying the task of the counsellor as a facilitator with the task of helping the individual or family to contain anxiety, resolve conflict and process emotions, facilitates the thinking processes necessary to enable good decision-making.

McConkie-Rosell and Sullivan (1999) discuss non-directiveness and consider that the idea does not have guiding theoretical principles. Using ideas similar to those in this book, they also use Lazarus and Folkman's Theory of Stress and Coping (1984), but propose that the concept of empowerment be used to help the individual. They consider that empowerment incorporates non-directiveness and is directed to enhancing individual autonomy and effective counselling interventions. They use four specific components of empowerment in relationship to genetic counselling: self-efficacy, developing skills, involvement with others and the development of a critical consciousness (Gutierrez, 1994). Their view is that 'there is a need to develop genetic counselling intervention models that are theory based, incorporate the value of non-directiveness and encompass the complex educational and counselling components that uniquely comprise genetic counselling'. Their aim is to transfer control to the individual and to enhance their resources and ability to express and act upon their goals and desires. Further the genetic counselling interventions would be designed to reduce anxiety, enhance control and mastery and increase understanding (which is in keeping with the thrust of the idea developed in this book).

The struggle to find a framework for the interview in medical genetics is reflected by a number of authors who have put forward ideas to inform clinical practice. Diekman-Tapon (1999) has suggested an Object Relations Family Therapy as a model and Eunpu (1997) a Systemically-Based Technique. A shared decision-making model has been espoused by other authors (Elwyn et al., 2000) where both the patient and counsellor are involved in investigation and exploration, jointly understanding the story and each other. This means both would have responsibility for management decisions, diagnostic pathways and investigations.

The view taken in this book is that *the practice* of genetic counselling defines its identity and the questions can then be directed to how it is best performed. The discussion is moving towards what actually goes on in a genetic counselling consultation and what is the role of the counsellor? With particular reference to pre-symptomatic testing, Soldan et al. (2000) describe the tasks and process of the interview as follows: clarification of the individual's understanding; consideration of the effect of knowledge and exploration of usual coping resource and style; education and informing; reflection of the feelings before decision-making. These areas will necessitate what Sarangi et al. (2003) describe as the counsellor changing the footing to perform these different tasks; shifting from questioning to listening, from empathising to challenging and from the particular to the bigger picture. The ensuing discussion may include information-giving and facilitating psychological adjustment. Soldan et al. (2000) question the usefulness of the cognitive decision-making model to the presymptomatic testing arena and advocate the use of models of human emotions and behaviour. They consider these would help foster emotional insight and understanding, a prerequisite in the decision-making process.

Reflective frames

In their discussion Sarangi et al. (2003) question the nature of genetic counselling and ask is it primarily an educative endeavour, aimed at maintaining psychological adjustment? Further, is it an attempt to impose a method on the decision-making process, or to ensure a high uptake for predictive testing, or, finally, client led?

Adopting a different approach, Sarangi et al. (2004) have focused on the discourse analysis of interviews exploring what actually goes on in the consulting room. In their paper 'Initiating reflective frames in counselling for Huntington's disease', they consider that the counsellor is adopting a non-directive stance by constructing 'reflective frames'. These invite the patients to discuss their feelings and encourage them to span their past, present and hypothetical future. They identify six categories of counsellors' reflective questions: non-specific usually used at the beginning; awareness of anxiety about the disorder for the patient and their family; decisions and how they are arrived at; the impact of the result; how the patient would disseminate the result and others to include coping and family dynamics. In their analysis of a series of interviews they found that the questions clustered at particular times in a Huntington's disease protocol. In the early stages, the questions focused on raising issues and concentrated on the decision-making process; in the later stages the focus shifted to the impact of a result. One of the techniques used by the counsellor would be to invite the patient to imagine various scenarios in the future, contrasting over time and comparing different people's reactions. Examples would include, 'How would you feel if you had a positive result to your test?' 'Can you imagine having a positive result?' and vice versa. 'Who would you speak to first when you have your result?' 'Who would be most upset about the result, you or your wife?' This type of interviewing is well established in family therapy where imagining, contrasting, or using a hierarchy, can help clarify and define and is described in Chapter 6. Imagining how things might be requires a considerable degree of personal security and with insecure individuals the counsellor may need to make the scenario more specific to be less threatening. For example, 'Let's imagine you've had your test result and the result is negative, you go home and you are thinking about it all, what sort of things would you be thinking and saying to your partner?'

The struggle with the concept of non-directiveness is not confined to genetic counselling – family therapists and psychoanalysts have struggled with what they call neutrality, their term for not influencing the patient. The genetic counsellor does not need to be a family therapist but, it may be useful to explore and understand the development in thinking in the field of family therapy and psychoanalysis.

Developments in family therapy from neutrality to curiosity, the use of narrative and a 'not-knowing' position

In 1980 a group of four psychoanalysts, known as the Milan Team, put forward ground breaking systemic guidelines for conducting an interview in a paper entitled 'Hypothesising-circularity-neutrality: Three guidelines for the conductor of a session' (Selvini-Palazzoli et al., 1980). That paper presented ways of questioning which started from a systemic framework and explored different view points around an event, idea or feeling as described in more detail in Chapter 6 under circular questioning. Cecchin, one member of the group, revisited the theme of neutrality in 1987 stating how he considered that it was impossible to be neutral as all behaviour, including language, is biased in some way. He pointed out that the idea behind neutrality had not been understood and, as in genetic counselling, in an attempt to be neutral, some professionals had adopted a position of non-involvement so appearing cold and aloof. Further, he explained that the real intent was to avoid considering any one position as more correct than another. To counter the difficulty, Cecchin proposed an attitude of curiosity, which would result in a constant search for more and more understanding, for multiple perspectives of the same event, relationship or story, etc. In exploring multiple perspectives the counsellor would not be attached to any particular view, but would explore many view points confirming that there is no one truth, but rather, different ways of looking at or understanding an issue. For example, applying the idea of curiosity to genetic counselling, an individual might be telling a story of how a family rift has developed around the genetic problem. With an attitude of curiosity, the counsellor might ask how that had come about, what else was happening in the family at the time, but, most importantly, how did other people view the rift and what effect did it have on relationships? Other questions might include asking who was most upset and how did others react to the upset? In asking these questions the counsellor is inviting the individual to explore and review the story which has been held for some time. The counsellor has not accepted that there was only one way of viewing the rift but, proposed that multiple perspectives might exist.

Family therapists have always been interested in the relationship patterns around an event and consider that by focusing on the relationship patterns around an event, rather than the event itself, new ways of thinking are triggered.

This idea of curiosity has been demonstrated by many of the examples given in this book.

Family therapy moved from an interest in the different relationship patterns or view points to a focus on the story an individual has about relationships – hence narrative therapy. The family therapist is interested in the multiple stories which can be told about the family and its relationships over time. Narrative therapy is particularly interesting as it links with attachment theory and the way an individual tells their story. In attachment theory, the more securely attached individual is able to tell a story with appropriate emotionality and from a position of self-reflection. In the same way in family therapy, the counsellor's curiosity, in the form of on-going interest and desire to understand, facilitates self-reflection and different thinking to allow for multiple perspectives and stories to be evolved. Again, the purpose is not solely to find a more 'healing story' but to stimulate different ways of thinking. In the earlier chapters considerable emphasis has been placed on the importance of facilitating self-reflection in the patient or family. In particular, it is important in genetic counselling for the patient to be able to reflect on their genetic story and the relationships around it. In many ways genetic counselling could be seen as a special form of narrative therapy.

Narrative therapy also links with modern psychoanalysis and, as Larner (2000) has pointed out, the narrative journey is undertaken in the context of a two-person relationship. The term inter-subjectivity is used to describe this conversation between two people. The modern analyst no longer behaves like a blank screen interpreting from a position of expertise but, like the family therapist, is interested in developing a conversation where the analyst is collaborating with their patient to jointly develop an understanding together (referred to earlier as co-construction in Chapter 4). These ideas from family therapy and psychoanalysis are in sympathy with the aim of genetic counselling where the collaborative conversation is directed towards helping the patient develop a narrative about their personal genetic inheritance.

The most recent development in both family therapy and psychoanalysis is the adoption of a position of 'not-knowing'. This is not a position of ignorance, but means that the counsellor is constantly open, not interpreting or intervening too early, waiting for the ideas to develop in the individual or family. For Anderson and Goolishian (1992) a therapeutic conversation occurs when there is a 'not-knowing' stance, encouraging a conversation around the problem that allows new meanings to emerge. The position of 'not-knowing' allows curiosity and exploration for new ideas to develop. Anderson (2001) clarifies the meaning of 'not-knowing' in stating that it refers to the therapist's intent and position or attitude, with a willingness to remain open to question and change. Further, she explains how 'not-knowing' has been misunderstood to imply a therapist lacks knowledge, feigns ignorance, withholds knowledge, avoids suggestions, or forgets what she knows. The central point is that it is not a technique or an expertise but, an ethical position. Bott (2001) picks up this theme saying that there are no therapeutic experts in the traditional sense of holding a privileged story. However, there is an art in developing a conversation where problems are understood within the context of meaning generated through language. Further, he describes the expert practitioner as having notions of 'conversation', 'collaboration' and 'curiosity' while taking the position of 'not-knowing'.

It is interesting to see how all these writers whether from family therapy or psychoanalysis are addressing the same problem as genetic counselling. The last author, Bott, brings us back to the meaning of the 'expert practitioner' and in genetic counselling that does not refer to having correct genetic information. Rather, it means being the psychological facilitator, in the service of the patient developing self-reflective thinking. For the genetic counsellor, the struggle will be to straddle the divide of knowing and giving genetic information only then to behave differently in order to explore and collaborate in a conversation 'not-knowing'. The latter position shifts away from the professional knowing facts to a situation where the counsellor is the learner who wants to understand the individual's story and way of being. Keats (1958) uses the term 'negative capability' to describe 'When man is capable of being in uncertainties, mysteries, doubts, without any irritable reaching after facts and reason'. In counselling, a psychological space can be created where there is no fixed view point but rather, an open conversation between two people trying to understand different meanings, view points or ways of thinking about an issue.

This consideration of the concept of non-directiveness in the context of ideas from family therapy and psychoanalysis has ended appropriately with the importance of the professional and the client working together. This is very much in keeping with the ideas about genetic counselling developed throughout in this book where the importance of the relationship between the counsellor and patient has been emphasised. Within that framework the task of the counsellor is to be both informer and facilitator, whilst taking an attitude of non-directiveness (of not influencing the decision), where the understanding of non-directiveness is of being constantly open, always seeking to understand further, so exploring and opening the discussion.

The counsellor can be viewed as an experienced companion who is attempting to accompany the patient on a journey of understanding, constantly trying to understand and clarify the patient's intention. As we have discussed earlier, understanding the intention is to be attuned to the individual which the author believes is professional intimacy.

Concluding comments

This book has worked from the premise of finding a language to describe and understand what genetic counselling is in practice. It has paralleled the genetic interview by putting forward a body of information before moving to exploring the meaning of its impact. It offers macro- and micro-skills and takes the view that a theoretical underpinning is essential to understand the meaning and consequently places genetic counselling within the frame of psychological stress. The theory explains general principles of the behaviour of individuals and families who are seeking counselling. Attachment theory explains the individual differences in approach and reactions and helps the counsellor consider the nature of the professional relationship. The general principles of psychotherapy and family therapy flesh out the interview principles with micro-skills which are specific to the tasks of genetic counselling.

As a profession genetic counselling has asked questions and debated 'what is genetic counselling?' Is it now time for the profession to clearly state genetic counselling is what genetic counsellors do? Whereas there is an overall framework it will not have a fixed format as it will vary depending on the interaction of the individual and the nature of the disorder. However, it is clear that it is not genetics plus counselling but an active form of interviewing which is specific to a genetic counselling consultation, focused on the task with a need for a particular delicacy.

References

Ainsworth, M., Blehar, M., Waters, E. and Wall, S. (1978). *Patterns of Attachment*, Hillsdale, New Jersey: Erlbaum.

Anderson, H. (2001). Postmodern collaborative and person-centred therapies: what would Carl Rogers say? *Journal of Family Therapy*, 23, 339–360.

Anderson, H. and Goolishian, H. (1992). The client is the expert: a not-knowing approach to therapy. In *Therapy as Social Construction*, eds. S. Mcnamee and K. Gergen, London: Sage.

Antley, R.M. (1979). The genetic counsellor as facilitator of the counsellee's decision process. In *Genetic Counseling: Facts, Values and Norms*, eds. A.M. Capron, M. Lappe, F.R. Murray, T.M. Powledge, S.B. Twiss and D. Bergsma, New York: Alan R. Liss, pp. 137–168.

Archer, S. (1993). Shame, guilt and counterfeiting. *Journal of the British Association of Psychotherapists*, 24, 36–61.

Asen, E. and Jones, E. (2000). *Systemic Couple Therapy and Depression*, London and New York: Karnac.

Ashcroft, R. (1999). Genetic information and 'genetic identity'. In *Genetic Information and 'Genetic Identity'*, eds. A.K. Thompson and R. Chadwick, New York: Kluwer Academic/Plenum Publishers.

Bateson, G. (1973). *Steps to an Ecology of Mind*, St Albans: Paladin.

Baum, A., Friedman, A.L. and Zakawski, S.G. (1997). Stress and genetic testing for disease risk. *Health Psychology*, 16, 8–20.

Berkenstadt, M., Shiloh, S., Gargai, G., Katznelson, MB.-M. and Goldman, B. (1999). Perceived personal control (ppc): a new concept in measuring outcome of genetic counseling. *American Journal of Medical Genetics*, 82, 53–59.

Biesecker-Bowles, B. (1998). Future directions in genetic counseling: practical and ethical considerations. *Kennedy Institute Ethics Journal*, 8, 145–160.

Binedell, J., Soldan, J.R., Scourfield, J. and Harper, P.S. (1996). Huntington's disease predictive testing: the case for an assessment approach to requests from adolescents. *Journal Medical Genetics*, 33, 912–915.

Bion, W.R. (1959). 'Attacks on linking'. *International Journal of Psychoanalysis*, 40, 308–315.

Bion, W.R. (1962). Learning from experience. In *Seven Servants*, New York: Aronson.

Bloch, M., Fahy, M., Fox, S. and Hayden, M.R. (1989). Predictive testing for Huntington's disease: ll. Demographic characteristics, life-style patterns, attitudes and psychosocial assessments of the first 51 test candidates. *American Journal of Medical Genetics*, 32, 217–224.

Bloch, M., Adam, S., Fuller, B., Kremer, B., Welch, J.P., Wiggins, S., Whyte, P., Huggins, M., Theilmann, J. and Hayden, M.R. (1993). Diagnosis of Huntington disease: a model for the stages of psychological response based on experience of predictive testing program. *American Journal of Medical Genetics*, 47, 368–374.

Bordin, E.S. (1982). A working alliance based model of supervision. *The Counselling Psychologist*, 11, 35–42.

Bosco, A.F. (2000). Caring for the care-giver: the benefit of a peer supervision group. *Journal of Genetic Counseling*, 9, 425–430.

Bott, D. (2001). Client-centred therapy and family therapy: a review and commentary. *Journal of Family Therapy*, 23, 361–377.

Bowen, M. (1978). *Family Therapy in Clinical Practice*, New York: Jason Aronson.

Bowlby, J. (1973). *Attachment and Loss, Vol. 2, Separation, Anxiety and Anger*, New York: Basic Books.

Bowlby, J. (1979). *The Making and Breaking of Affectional Bonds*, London: Tavistock.

Bradbury, E. (1993). Psychological approaches to children and adolescents with disfigurement: a review of the literature. *Association of Child Psychology and Psychiatry Review & Newsletter*, 15, 1–5.

Brain, K., Soldan, J., Sampson, J. and Gray, J. (2003). Genetic counselling protocols for hereditary non-polyposis colorectal cancer: a survey of UK regional genetics centres. *Clinical Genetics*, 63, 198–204.

Brantley, H. and Clifford, E. (1979). Cognitive, self-concept and body image measurements on normal, cleft and obese adolescents. *Cleft Palate Journal*, 16, 177–182.

Bretherton, I. (1991). Pouring new wine into old bottles: the social self as internal working model. In *Self Processes and Development*, eds. M. Gunner and L. Sroufe, Hillsdale, New Jersey: Erlbaum.

Brewin, T.B. (1991). Three ways of giving bad news. *Lancet*, 337, 1207–1209.

Buckman, R. (1992). *How to Break Bad News*, London: Pan Macmillan.

Byng-Hall, J. (1995a). Myths and legends about security. In *Rewriting Family Scripts*, New York and London: Guildford Press.

Byng-Hall, J. (1995b). Creating a family science base: some implications of attachment theory for family therapy. *Family Process*, 34(1), 45–58.

Canadian Paediatric Society, Bioethics Committee (2003). Guidelines for genetic testing of healthy children. *Paediatrics and Child Health*, 8, 42–45.

Carter, E. and McGoldrick, M. (1989). *The Expanded Family Life Cycle*, 3rd edn, Boston: Allyn and Baco.

Cecchin, G. (1987). Hypothesising, circularity and neutrality revisited: an invitation to curiosity. *Family Process*, 26, 405–413.

Chapman, E. (2002). Ethical dilemmas in testing for late onset conditions: reactions to testing and perceived impact on other family members. *Journal of Genetic Counseling*, 11, 351–367.

Chasseguet-Smirgel, J. (1985). *The Ego Ideal*, London: Free Association.

Clarke, A. (1991). Is non-directive counselling possible? *Lancet*, 335, 1145–1147.

Clarke, A. and Flinter, F. (1996). The genetic testing of children: a clinical perspective. In *The Troubled Helix: Social and Psychological Implications of the New Human Genetics*, eds. T. Marteau and M. Richards, Cambridge, New York: Cambridge University Press.

Clarkeburn, H. (2000). Parental duties and untreatable genetic conditions. *Journal Medical Ethics*, 26, 400–403.

Codori, A.M. and Brandt, J. (1994). Psychological costs and benefits of predictive testing for Huntington's disease. *American Journal of Medical Genetics*, 54, 174–184.

Codori, A.M., Slavney, P.R., Young, C., Miglioretti, D.L. and Brandt, J. (1997). Predictor of psychological adjustment to genetic testing for Huntington's disease. *Health Psychology*, 16, 36–50.

Cohen, S. and Lazarus, R.S. (1979). Coping with the stresses of illness. In *Health Psychology: A Handbook*, eds. G.C. Stone, F. Cohen and N.E. Adler, San Francisco: Jossey-Bass, pp. 217–254.

Condon, W.S. (1984). Communication and empathy. In *Empathy II*, eds. J. Lichtenberg, M. Bornstein and D. Silver, Hillsdale, New Jersey: Analytic Press.

Counselman, E.F. and Gumpert, P. (1993). Psychotherapy supervision in small leader-led groups. *Group*, 17, 25–32.

Craufurd, D. and Tyler, A. (1992). Predictive testing for Huntington's disease: protocol of the Huntington's prediction consortium. *Journal of Medical Genetics*, 29, 915–918.

Craufurd, D., Dodge, A., Kerzin-Storrar, L. and Harris, R. (1989). Uptake of presymptomatic predictive testing for Huntington's disease. *Lancet*, 2, 603–605.

Craufurd, D., Binchy, A. and Evans, G. (1997). Uptake and impact of predictive testing – a comparison of breast-ovarian cancer and Huntington's disease. 5th European meeting on psychosocial aspects of genetics 1996 September 26–28th; Rome, Italy (Abstracts). *Genetic Counselling*, 8, 147–186.

Croyle, R.T., Smith, K.R., Botkin, J.R., Baty, B. and Nash, J. (1997). Psychological responses to the BRCA1 mutation testing: preliminary findings. *Health Psychology*, 16, 63–72.

Dennett, D.C. (1983). Styles of mental representation. *Proceedings of the Aristotelian Society.* London: Aristotelian Society, pp. 213–226.

Diekman-Tapon, D. (1999). Case report: object relations family therapy as a model for genetic counselling. *Journal of Genetic Counselling*, 8, 235–246.

Dozier, M., Cue, K. and Barnett, L. (1994). Clinicians as caregivers: role of attachment organisation in treatment. *Journal of Consulting and Clinical Psychology*, 62, 793–800.

Easterbrook, J.A. (1959). The effects of emotion on cue utilisation and organisation of behaviour. *Psychological Review*, 66, 183–201.

Elliot, T.S. (1944). *Four Quartets*, London: Faber and Faber.

Elwyn, G., Gray, J. and Clarke, A. (2000). Shared decision making and non-directiveness in genetic counselling. *Journal of Medical Genetics*, 37, 135–138.

Engel, G.L. (1961). Is grief a disease? A challenge for medical research. *Psychosomatic Medicine*, 23, 18–22.

Engel, G.L. (1962). *Psychological Development in Health and Disease*, Philadelphia: W.B. Saunders.

Erikson, E.H. (1950). *Childhood and Society*, New York: Norton and London.

Eunpu, D.L. (1997). Systemic-based psychotherapeutic techniques in genetic counselling. *Journal of Genetic Counseling*, 6, 1–20.

Evans, C. and Street, E. (2003). Genetic counseling and the family system. In *Nature Encyclopedia of Human Genome*, London and New York: Macmillan and Nature Publishing Group.

Evans, D.G.R., Maher, E.R., Maclead, R., Davies, D.R. and Craufurd, D. (1997). Uptake of genetic testing for cancer predisposition – ethical issues. *Journal of Medical Genetics*, 34, 746–749.

Evers-Kiebooms, G., Swerts, A. and Van den Berghe, H. (1988). Psychological aspects of amniocentesis: anxiety feelings in three different risk groups. *Clinical Genetics*, 33, 196–206.

Evers-Kiebooms, G., Swerts, A., Cassiman, J.J. and Van Den Berghe, H. (1989). The motivation of at risk individuals and their partners in deciding for and against predictive testing for Huntington's disease. *Clinical Genetics*, 35, 29–40.

Fajardo, B. (1987). Parenting a damaged child: mourning, regression and disappointment. *Psychoanalytic Review*, 74, 19–43.

Farrer, L.A. (1986). Suicide and attempted suicide in Huntingdon's disease: implications for preclinical testing of persons at risk. *American Journal of Medical Genetics*, 24, 305–311.

Field, T.M. and Vegha-Lahr, N. (1984). Early interactions between infants with cran-iofacial abnormalities and their mothers. *Infant Behaviour and Development*, 7, 527–530.

Folkman, S. (1984). Personal control and stress and coping processes: a theoretical analysis. *Journal of Personality and Social Psychology*, 48, 839–852.

Folkman, S. and Lazarus, R.S. (1985). If it changes, it must be process: a study of emotion and coping during three stages of a college examination. *Journal of Personality and Social Psychology*, 48, 150–170.

Fonagy, P. (1994). The theory and practice of resilience. *Journal of Child Psychology and Psychiatry*, 35, 231–257.

Fonagy, P. (1995). Attachment, the reflective self and borderline states. In *Attachment Theory: Social Development and Clinical Perspectives*, eds. S. Goldberg, R. Muir and J. Kerr, Hillsdale, New Jersey: Analytic Press.

France, L., Gray, J., Elwyn, G., Tischkowitz, M., Brain, K., Sampson, J., Anglim, C., Clarke, A., Parsons, E., Sweetland, H., Mansel, R., Barrett-Lee, P. and Harper, P. (1999). Genetic testing considerations in breast cancer patients. *Journal of Genetic Counseling*, 8, 289–299.

Fraser, F.C. (1974). Genetic counseling. *American Journal of Human Genetics*, 15, 1–10.

Fraser, F.C. (1979). Degree of directiveness. In *Genetic Counseling*, eds. H.A. Lubs and F. de la Cruz, New York: Raven Press.

Freud, S. (1937). *Analysis Terminable and Interminable, S.E. 23*, London: Hogarth and Institute of Psycho-Analysis.

Goffman, E. (1963). *Stigma: Notes on the Management of Spoiled Identity*, Ealewood Cliffs, New Jersey: Prentice-Hall.

Gordon, R. (1965). The concept of projective identification. *Journal of Analytic Psychology*, 10, 127–149.

Green, J. and Statham, H. (1996). Psychosocial aspects of prenatal screening and diagnosis. In *The Troubled Helix: Social and Psychological Implications of the New Human Genetics*, eds. T. Marteau and M. Richards, Cambridge, New York: Cambridge University Press.

Gutierrez, L.M. (1994). Beyond coping: an empowerment perspective on stressful life events. *Journal of Sociology and Social Welfare*, 21, 201–219.

Harper, P.S. (1997). Presymptomatic testing for late-onset genetic disorders: lessons from Huntington's disease. In *Genetics, Society and Clinical Practise*, eds. P.S. Harper and A.J. Clarke, Oxford and Herndon VA: Bios Scientific.

Harwood, R.L., Miller, J.G. and Irizarry, N.L. (1995). *Culture and Attachment: Perceptions of the Child in Context*, New York: Guilford.

Hawkins, P. and Shohet, R. (1989). *Supervision in the Helping Professions: An Individual, Group and Organisational Approach*, Milton Keynes: Open University.

Heard, D. (1982). Family systems and the attachment dynamic. *Journal of Family Therapy*, 4, 99–116.

Heimann, P. (1950). On countertransference. *International Journal of Psycho-Analysis*, 31, 81–84.

Hiller, E. and Rosenfield, J.M. (2000). The Experience of leader-led peer supervision: genetic counselors' perspectives. *Journal of Genetic Counseling*, 9, 399–410.

Hoeksma, J.B. and Koomen, H. (1991). *Development of Early Mother and Child Interaction*, Amsterdam: Pro Lingua.

Holmes, J. (1996). *Attachment, Intimacy, Autonomy: Using Attachment Theory in Adult Psychotherapy*, Northville, New Jersey: Jason Aronson.

Holmes, J. (2001). *The Search for the Secure Base*, Hove and New York: Brunner Routledge.

Holmes, J. (2004). Disorganised attachment and borderline personality disorder: a clinical perspective. *Attachment & Human Development*, 6(2), 181–190.

Horowitz, M., Sundin, E., Zanko, A. and Lauer, R. (2001). Coping with grim news from genetic tests. *Psychosomatics*, 42, 100–105.

Howes, C. (1999). Attachment relationships in the context of multiple caregivers. In *Handbook of Attachment: Theory, Research and Clinical Applications*, eds. J. Cassidy and R. Shaver, New York and London: Guilford.

Hsai, Y.E. (1979). The genetic counselling as information giver. In *Risk Communication and Decision Making in Genetic Counselling*, eds. C.J.R. Curry, S. Packman, S. Sherman and B.D. Hall, New York: Alan R. Liss, pp. 168–186.

Janis, I.L. (1958). *Psychological Stress. Psychoanalytic and Behavioural Studies of Surgical Patients*, London: Chapman and Hall.

Janis, I.L. and Mann, L. (1977). *Decision Making; A Psychological Analysis of Conflict*, New York: Free Press.

Jones, E. (1993). *Family Systems Therapy: Development in the Milan-Systemic Therapies*, Chichester: John Wiley.

Juengst, E.T. (1999). Genetic testing and the moral dynamics of family life. *Public Understand Science*, 8, 193–205.

Karp, J., Brown, K.L., Sullivan, M.D. and Massie, M.J. (1999). The prophylactic mastectomy dilemma: a support group for women at high genetic risk for breast cancer. *Journal of Genetic Counseling*, 8, 163–173.

Kash, K.M., Holland, J.C., Halper, M.S. and Miller, D.G. (1992). Psychological distress and surveillance behaviours of women with a family history of breast cancer. *Journal of National Cancer Institute*, 84, 24–30.

Keats, J. (1958). Letters of John Keats, No. 11, ed. H.E. Rollin, Cambridge [Mass]: Harvard University Press.

Kenen, R., Smith, A.C.M., Watkins, C. and Zuber-Pittore, C. (2000). To use or not to use: the prenatal genetic technology/worry conundrum. *Journal of Genetic Counseling*, 9, 203–217.

Kennedy, A.L. (2000a). Supervision of practicing genetic counselors: an overview of models. *Journal of Genetic Counseling*, 9, 379–390.

Kennedy, A.L. (2000b). A leader-led supervision group as a model for practicing genetic counselors. *Journal of Genetic Counseling*, 9, 391–397.

Kessler, S. (1980). The psychological paradigm shift in genetic counseling. *Social Biology*, 27, 167–185.

Kessler, S. (1984). Psychological aspects of genetic counseling. III. Management of guilt and shame. *American Journal Medical Genetics*, 17, 673–697.

Kessler, S. (1987). Psychiatric complications for testing for Huntington's disease. *American Journal Medical Genetics*, 57, 212–219.

Kessler, S. (1988). Invited essay on the psychological aspects of genetic counseling. V. Preselection: a family coping strategy in Huntington's disease. *American Journal of Medical Genetics*, 31, 617–621.

Kessler, S. (1992a). Psychological aspects of genetic counselling. VII. Thoughts on directiveness. *Journal of Genetic Counseling*, 1, 9–17.

Kessler, S. (1992b). Psychological aspects of genetic counselling. VIII. Suffering and countertransference. *Journal of Genetic Counseling*, 1, 303–308.

Kessler, S. (1993). Forgotten person in the Huntingdon disease family. *American Journal of Medical Genetics*, 48, 145–150.

Kessler, S. (1997). Psychological aspects of genetic counseling. XI. Non-directiveness revisited. *American Journal of Medical Genetics*, 72, 164–171.

Kessler, S. (2000). Closing thoughts on supervision. *Journal of Genetic Counseling*, 9, 431–434.

Klein, M. (1952). The emotional life of the infant. In *Envy and Gratitude and Other Works*, London: Hogarth.

Kohut, H. (1971). *The Analysis of the Self*, New York: International Universities Press.

Kozlowska, K. and Hanney, L. (2002). The network perspective: an integration of attachment and family system theories. *Family Process*, 41(3), 285–312.

Lansdown, R., Lloyd, J. and Hunter, J. (1991). Facial deformity in childhood: severity and psychological adjustment. *Child: Care, Health and Development*, 17, 165–171.

Larner, G. (2000). Towards a common ground in psychoanalysis and family therapy: on knowing not to know. *Journal of Family Therapy*, 22, 61–82.

Lax, R.F. (1972). Some aspects of the interaction between mother and impaired child: mother's narcissistic trauma. *Internal Journal of Psycho-Analysis*, 53, 339–344.

Lazarus, R.S. and Folkman, S. (1984). *Stress, Appraisal and Coping*, New York: Springer.

Lerman, C. (1997). Psychological aspects of genetic testing: introduction to the special issue. *Health Psychology*, 16, 3–8.

Lerman, C., Trock, B., Rimer, B.K., Jepson, C., Brody, D. and Boyce, A. (1991). Psychological side effects of breast cancer screening. *Health Psychology*, 10, 259–267.

Lerman, C., Kash, K. and Stefanek, M. (1994). Younger women at an increased risk for breast cancer: perceived risk, psychological well-being and surveillance behaviour. *Monographs: National Cancer Institute*, 16, 171–176.

Lerman, C., Seay, J., Balshem, A. and Audrain, J. (1995). Interest in genetic testing among first-degree relatives of breast cancer relatives. *American Journal of Medical Genetics*, 57, 385–392.

Lerman, C., Narod, S., Schulman, K., Hughes, C., Gomez-Caminero, A. and Bonney, G. (1996). BRCA1 testing in families with hereditary breast-ovarian cancer: a prospective study of patient decision-making and outcomes. *Journal of the American Medical Association*, 275, 1885–1892.

Lerman, C., Schwartz, M.D., Lin, T.H., Hughes, C., Narod, S. and Lynch, H.T. (1997). The influence of psychological distress on use of genetic testing for cancer risk. *Journal of Consulting and Clinical Psychology*, 65, 414–420.

Lerman, C., Hughes, C., Lemon, S.J., Main, D., Snyder, C., Durham, C., Narod, S. and Lynch, H.T. (1998). What you don't know can hurt you: adverse psychological effects in members of BRCA1-linked and BRCA2-linked families who decline genetic testing. *Journal of Clinical Oncology*, 16, 1650–1654.

Likhite, M.L. (2000). The interface between countertransference and projective identification in a case presented to peer supervision. *Journal of Genetic Counseling*, 9, 417–424.

Lippman, A. (1999). Embodied knowledge and making sense of prenatal diagnosis. *Journal of Genetic Counseling*, 8, 255–274.

Machin, L. (2001). Exploring a framework for understanding the range of response to loss, a study of clients receiving bereavement counselling, *Unpublished Ph.D. thesis*, Keele University, UK.

Machin, L. and Spall, B. (2004). Mapping grief: a study in practise using a quantitative and qualitative approach to exploring and addressing the range of responses to loss. *Counselling and Psychotherapy Research*, 4, 9–17.

Main, M. (1995). Recent studies in attachment: overview with selected implications for clinical work. In *Attachment Theory: Social, Developmental and Clinical Perspectives*, eds. S. Goldberg, R. Muir and J. Kerr, Hillsdale, New Jersey: Analytic Press.

Main, M. and Goldwyn, S. (1995). Interview based adult attachment classification: related to infant-mother and infant-father attachment. *Developmental Psychology*, 19, 227–239.

McConkie-Rosell, A. and Sullivan, J.A. (1999). Genetic counselling-stress, coping and the empowerment perspective. *Journal of Genetic Counseling*, 8, 345–357.

McGoldrick, M. and Gerson, R. (1985). *Genograms in Family Assessments*, New York and London: W.W. Norton.

McGregor, F. (1970). Social and psychological implications of dentofacial disfigurement. *Angle Orthodontist*, 40, 231–233.

Meiser, B. and Dunn, S. (2000). Psychological impact of genetic testing for Huntington's disease: an update of the literature. *Journal of Neurology, Neurosurgery and Psychiatry*, 69, 574–578.

Meiser, B., Gleeson, M.A. and Tucker, K.M. (2000). Psychological impact of genetic testing for adult-onset disorders. *Medical Journal of Australia*, 172, 125–129.

Meissen, G.J., Myers, R.H., Mastromauro, C.A., Koroshetz, W., Klinger, K.W., Farrer, L.A., Watkins, P.A., Gusella, J.F., Bird, E.D. and Martin, J.B. (1988). Predictive testing for Huntington's disease with the use of a linked DNA marker. *New England Journal of Medicine*, 318, 535–542.

Meltzoff A. and Gopnik N. (1993). The role of limitation in understanding persons and developing a theory of mind. In *Understanding Other Minds*, eds. S. Baron-Cohen, H. Tager-Flusberg and D. Cohen, New York: Oxford University Press, pp. 335–366.

Michie, S. (1996). Predictive genetic testing in children: paternalism or empiricism. In *The Troubled Helix: Social and Psychological Implications of the New Human Genetic*, eds. T. Marteau and M. Richards, Cambridge, New York: Cambridge University Press.

Miller, S.M. and Morgan, C.E. (1983). Interacting effects of information and coping style in adapting to gynaecological stress: should the doctor tell all? *Journal of Personality and Social Psychology*, 45, 233–236.

Mollon, P. (1997). Supervision as a space for thinking. In *Supervision of Psychotherapy and Counselling: Making a Place to Think*, ed. G. Shipton, Buckingham: Open University Press.

Olsen, D.H., Russell, C.S. and Sprenkle, D.H. (1988). *Circumplex Model: Systemic Assessment and Treatment of Families*, New York: Haworth Press.

Park, J. (2004). Walking the tightrope: developing an attachment-based/relational curriculum for trainee psychotherapists. *Attachment and Human Development*, 6, 117–130.

Parkes, C.M. (2001). *Bereavement. Studies in Grief in Adult Life*, 3rd edn, Philadelphia: Taylor & Francis.

Pines, M. (1993). The world according to Kohut. *Journal of the British Association of Psychotherapists*, 25, 47–63.

Quill, T.E. and Townsend, P. (1991). Bad news: delivery, dialogue and dilemmas. *Archives of Internal Medicine*, 151, 463–468.

Richards, M. (1996). Families, kinship and genetics. In *The Troubled Helix: Social and Psychological Implications of the New Human Genetics*, eds. T. Marteau and M. Richards, Cambridge, New York: Cambridge University Press.

Roberts, C., Wass, V., Jones, R., Sarangi, S. and Gillett, A. (2003). A discourse analysis study of 'good' and 'poor' communication in an OSCE: a proposed new framework for teaching students. *Medical Education*, 37, 192–201.

Rogers C.R. (1957). The necessary and sufficient conditions for therapeutic personality change. *Journal of Consulting Psychology*, 21, 95–103.

Rolland, J.S. (1984). A psychosocial typology of chronic illness. *Family Systems Medicine*, 2, 245–262.

Rowland, J.H. (1990). Interpersonal resources: social support. In *Handbook of Psycho-oncology*, eds. J.C. Holland and J.H. Rowland, New York: Oxford University Press.

Rutter, M. (1987). Psychosocial resilience and protective mechanisms. In *Risk and Protection Factors in the Development of Psychopathology*, eds. S. Rolk, A. Master, D. Cicicchetti, K. Muechtelein and S. Weintraub, New York: Cambridge University Press.

Sarangi, S. (2000). Activity types, discourse types and interactional hybridity: the case of genetic counselling. In *Discourse and Social Life*, eds. S. Sarangi and M. Coultard, London: Longman.

Sarangi, S. and Clarke, A. (2002). Constructing an account by contrast in genetic counselling for childhood genetic testing. *Social Science and Medicine*, 54, 295–308.

Sarangi, S., Bennett, K., Howell, L. and Clarke, A. (2003). 'Relatively speaking': relativisation of genetic risk in counselling for predictive testing. *Health, Risk Society*, 5(2), 155–170.

Sarangi, S., Bennett, K., Howell, L., Clarke, A., Harper, P. and Gray, J. (2004). Initiation of reflective frames in counselling for Huntington's disease predictive testing. *Journal of Genetic Counseling*, 13(2), 129–150.

Selvini-Palazzoli, M., Boscolo, L., Cecchin, G. and Prata, G. (1980). Hypothesizing-circularity-neutrality: three guidelines for the conductor of the session. *Family Process*, 19, 3–12.

Shaw, W.C. (1981). Folklore surrounding facial deformity and the origins of facial prejudice. *British Journal of Plastic Surgery*, 34, 237–246.

Shiloh, S. (1996). Decision-making in the context of genetic risk. In *The Troubled Helix: Social and Psychological Implications of the New Human Genetics*, eds. T. Marteau and M. Richards, Cambridge, New York: Cambridge University Press.

Shiloh, S. and Saxe, L. (1989). Perception of recurrence risks by genetic counselees. *Psychology and Health*, 3, 45–61.

Shiloh, S., Berkenstadt, M., Meiran, N., Bat-Miriam-Katznelson, M. and Goldman, B. (1997). Mediating affects of perceived personal control in coping with a health threat: the case of genetic counseling. *Journal of Applied Social Psychology*, 27, 1146–1174.

Slade, A. (1999). Individual psychotherapy: an attachment perspective. In *Handbook of Attachment. Theory, Research and Clinical Applications*, eds. J. Cassidy and P.R. Shaver, New York and London: Guilford Press.

Soldan, J., Street, E., Gray, J., Binedell, J. and Harper, P. (2000). Psychological model for presymptomatic test interviews: lessons learned from Huntington's disease. *Journal of Genetic Counseling*, 9(1), 15–31.

Solnit, A.J. and Stark, M.H. (1961). Mourning and the birth of a defective child. *Psychoanalytic Study Child*, 16.

Stadler, M.P. and Mulvihill, J.J. (1998). Cancer risk assessment and genetic counseling in an academic medical center: consultants' satisfaction, knowledge and behavior in the first year. *Journal of Genetic Counseling*, 7, 279–297.

Street, E.C. (1994). *Counselling for Family Problems*, London: Sage.

Street, E.C. and Soldon, J. (1998). A conceptual framework for the psychosocial issues faced by families with genetic conditions. *Families Systems and Health*, 16, 217–231.

Tarnopolsky, A. (1995). Understanding countertransference. *Psychoanalytic Psychotherapy*, 9, 185–194.

Thewes, B., Meiser, B., Tucker, M. and Tucker, K. (2003). The unmet information and support needs of women with a family history of breast cancer: a descriptive survey. *Journal of Genetic Counseling*, 12, 61–76.

Tibben, A. (1993). *What is Knowledge but Grieving? On Psychological Effects of Presymptomatic DNA-Testing for Huntington's Disease (Dissertations)*, Rotterdam: University of Rotterdam.

Tibben, A., Vegter-vander Vlis, M., Neirmeijer, M.F., Vande Kamp, J.J.P., Roos, R.A.C., Rooijmans, H.G.M., Frets, P.G. and Verhage, F. (1990). Testing for Huntingdon's disease with support of all parties. *Lancet*, 335, 553.

Tibben, A., Neirmeijer, M.F., Roos, R.A.C., Vegter-vander Vlis, M., Frets, P.G., Vande Kamp, J.J. and Verhage, F. (1992). Understanding the low uptake of presymptomatic DNA testing in Huntingdon's disease. *Lancet*, 340, 1416.

Tibben, A., Tinman, R., Bannink, E.C. and Duivenvoorden, H.J. (1997). Three-year follow-up after presymptomatic testing for Huntingdon's disease in tested individuals and partners. *Health Psychology*, 16, 20–35.

Timberlake, E.M. (1985). Self-concept protection by children with physical differences. *Child and Adolescent Social Work Journal*, 2, 232–245.

Vernon, S.W., Gritz, E.R., Peterson, S.K., Amos, C.I., Perz, C.A., Baile, W.F. and Linch, P.M. (1997). Correlates of psychological distress in colorectal cancer patients undergoing genetic testing for hereditary colon cancer. *Health Psychology*, 16, 73–86.

Watzlawich, P., Weakland, J. and Fisch, R. (1974). *Change: Principles of Problem Formation and Resolution*, New York: W.W. Norton.

Weil, J. (2000). Introduction. *Journal of Genetic Counseling*, 9, 375–378.

Weil, J. (2003). Psychosocial genetic counselling in the post-non-directive era: a point of view. *Journal of Genetic Counseling*, 12, 199–211.

Wexler, N.S. (1979). Genetic 'Russian Roulette': the experience of being at risk of Huntington's disease. In *Genetic Counselling: Psychological Dimensions*, ed. S.J. Kessler, New York: Academic Press.

Wexler, N.S. (1992). The Tiresias Complex: Huntington's disease as a paradigm of testing for late-onset disorders. *Federation of American Societies for Experimental Biology Journal*, 6, 2820–2825.

White, K. (2004). Developing secure-enough base: teaching psychotherapists in training the relationship between attachment theory and clinical work. *Attachment and Human Development*, 6, 117–130.

Wiggins, S., Whyte, P., Huggins, M., Adm, S., Theilmann, J., Bloch, M., Sheps, S.B., Schechter, M.T. and Hayden, M.R. (1992). The psychological consequences of predictive testing for Huntington's disease. *The New England Journal of Medicine*, 327, 1401–1405.

Winnicott, D.W. (1965). *The Maturational Processes and the Facilitating Environment: Studies in the Theory of Emotional Development*, London: Hogarth and Institute of Psycho-Analysis.

Winnicott, D.W. (1971). *Playing and Reality*, London: Tavistock.

Winnicott, D.W. (1988). *Human Nature*, London: Free Association.

Wolf, N. (1990). *The Beauty Myth: How Images of Beauty Are Used against Women*, London: Chatto and Windus.

Wolff, G. and Jung, C. (1995). Non-directiveness and genetic counseling. *Journal of Genetic Counseling*, 4, 3–25.

Worden, J.W. (1991). *Grief Counselling and Grief Therapy*, London: Routledge.

Index

EDITOR: LEE JOHNSON

**OSPREY
MILITARY**

WARRIOR SERIES

NORMAN KNIGHT
950–1204AD

Text by
CHRISTOPHER GRAVETT
Colour plates by
CHRISTA HOOK

Published in 1993 by
Osprey Publishing Ltd
59 Grosvenor Street, London W1X 9DA
© Copyright 1993 Osprey Publishing Ltd

ISBN 1 85532 270 6

Filmset in Great Britain
Printed and bound in Great Britain by
Butler & Tanner Ltd, Frome and London

Dedication
For Jane, with thoughts of Jumièges.

Acknowledgements
I should like to thank the following for many hours of
useful discussion, argument and for advice: Andrew
Bodley, Chris Dobson, Ian Eaves, Brian Gilmour,
Jeremy Hall, Mark Harrison, Dr. David Nicolle and
Karen Watts.

Artist's Note
Readers may care to note that the original paintings
from which the colour plates in this book were
prepared are available for private sale. All
reproduction copyright whatsoever is retained by the
publisher. All enquiries should be addressed to:

Scorpio Gallery
PO Box 475
Hailsham
E. Sussex BN27 2SL

The publishers regret that they can enter into no
correspondence upon this matter.

Publisher's Note
Readers may wish to study this title in conjunction
with the following Osprey publications:

MAA 85	*Saxon, Viking and Norman Armies*
MAA 171	*Saladin and the Saracens*
MAA 89	*Byzantine Armies 886–1118*
MAA 75	*Armies of the Crusades*
MAA 231	*French Medieval Armies 1000–1300*
Elite 9	*The Normans*
Elite 3	*The Vikings*
Campaign 13	*Hastings 1066*

For a catalogue of all books published by Osprey Military
please write to:

**The Marketing Manager,
Consumer Catalogue Department,
Osprey Publishing Ltd,
Michelin House, 81 Fulham Road,
London SW3 6RB**